T0200389

Residential, Home and Community Aged Care
WORKBOOK
3rd edition

Carla Unicomb
RN, Bachelor of Health Science (Nursing), Graduate Certificate in VET,
Graduate Certificate in OHS, Certificate IV in Training and Assessment
Director, Training Beyond 2000

Wendy Bell
RN, Bachelor of Health Science (Nursing)
Certificate IV in Training and Assessment
Diploma of Dementia Care
Principal Trainer, Training Beyond 2000

Disclaimer:

These materials have been written to the latest version of the qualifications and units of competence. However, it is up to each individual registered training organisation to ensure that it is meeting the requirements of the latest version of the training package/units of competence.

ELSEVIER

ELSEVIER

Elsevier Australia. ACN 001 002 357
(a division of Reed International Books Australia Pty Ltd)
Tower 1, 475 Victoria Avenue, Chatswood, NSW 2067

Copyright 2024 Elsevier Australia.

Second Edition © 2018; First edition © 2016.

ISBN: 978-0-7295-4380-4

Notice

This publication has been carefully reviewed and checked to ensure that the content is as accurate and current as possible at time of publication. We would recommend, however, that the reader verify any procedures, treatments, drug dosages or legal content described in this book. Neither the author, the contributors nor the publisher assume any liability for injury and/or damage to persons or property arising from any error in or omission from this publication.

National Library of Australia Cataloguing-in-Publication Data

 A catalogue record for this book is available from the National Library of Australia

Content Strategist: Melinda McEvoy
Content Project Manager: Shravan Kumar
Edited by Margaret Trudgeon
Proofread by Tim Learner
Copyrights Coordinator: Deepika Gopal
Cover Designer: Lisa Petroff
Typeset by GW Tech
Printed in China by 1010 Printing International Limited
Last digit is the print number: 9   8   7   6   5   4   3   2   1

Contents

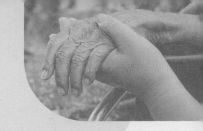

Preface

This workbook has been written to address the most current aged care training package requirements and is a resource to support the fifth edition of Scott, Webb and Kostelnick's *Long-Term Caring: Residential, Home and Community Aged Care* textbook.

Aimed at learners undertaking aged care qualifications, the workbook has been prepared after extensive consultation with aged care providers and considering feedback from past training participants. We especially acknowledge the contribution of Penny Kraemer, a registered pharmacist, who was the author of the chapter entitled 'Assist Clients with Medication'.

We would like to express our sincere thanks to Melinda McEvoy for her valuable support and suggestions in preparing the workbook.

Carla Unicomb
Wendy Bell

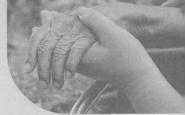

How to use this workbook

This workbook accompanies the fifth edition of Scott, Webb and Kostelnick's *Long-Term Caring: Residential, Home and Community Aged Care* textbook, published by Elsevier. The Workbook, Written Assessment, Practical Assessment, PowerPoint slides and Mapping have been written to cover the units of competence in Certificate III in Individual Support. The workbook can be used in face-to-face classroom presentation or in online learning setup.

The workbook should be used in conjunction with a registered training organisation's training and assessment plans, and can be customised and contextualised to satisfy the industry and the training organisation's requirements.

About the Authors

Carla Unicomb and Wendy Bell are registered nurses, both with over 40 years of nursing and vocational education and training experience.

Carla Unicomb is the Director of Training Beyond 2000 Pty Limited, an RTO specialising in aged care training since 2000. Carla has been serving the fraternity with her keen interest in health, safety, infection control and aged care sector.

Wendy Bell is the Principal Trainer with Training Beyond 2000 Pty Limited, specialising in training staff to work in the aged care sector. Wendy is passionate about every person receiving needs-based, person-centred quality care and having well-trained empathetic staff who will respond to their individual needs.

In preparing these learning materials, Carla and Wendy have drawn upon the resources they have developed in consultation with aged care providers over the past 18 years. The learning and assessment activities reflect real work-based contexts and provide the learner with the opportunity to demonstrate that they have the requisite knowledge and skills to competently perform their role in the community services and health industry.

Carla and Wendy are passionate about delivering high-quality training and assessment that allows learners to transfer knowledge and skills to their work environment. Their newly acquired knowledge and skills will assist the learner to deliver person-centred care that enhances the quality of life of the care recipient.

Contributor

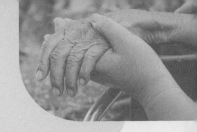

Penny Kraemer BPharm, MPS
Pharmacist, Port Macquarie, NSW, Australia

1

Unit CHCAGE013:
Work effectively in aged care

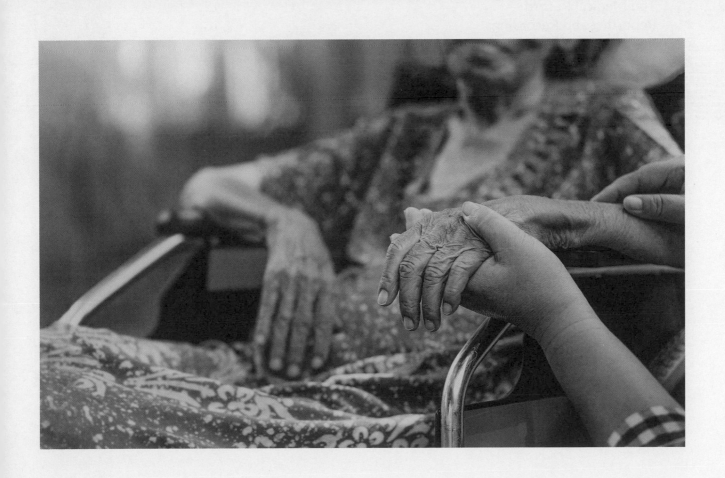

Table of Contents

INTRODUCTION

This workbook relates to the unit **CHCAGE013: Work effectively in aged care**. The workbook activities and final assessment tasks will enable you to:

- meet job role requirements
- work within organisational requirements
- work within an aged care context
- implement self-care strategies.

To prepare for this unit and the assessment activities, we recommend that you first read Chapter 1 of Scott, Webb and Kostelnick, 5th edition, **Health and aged care services in Australia and New Zealand**.

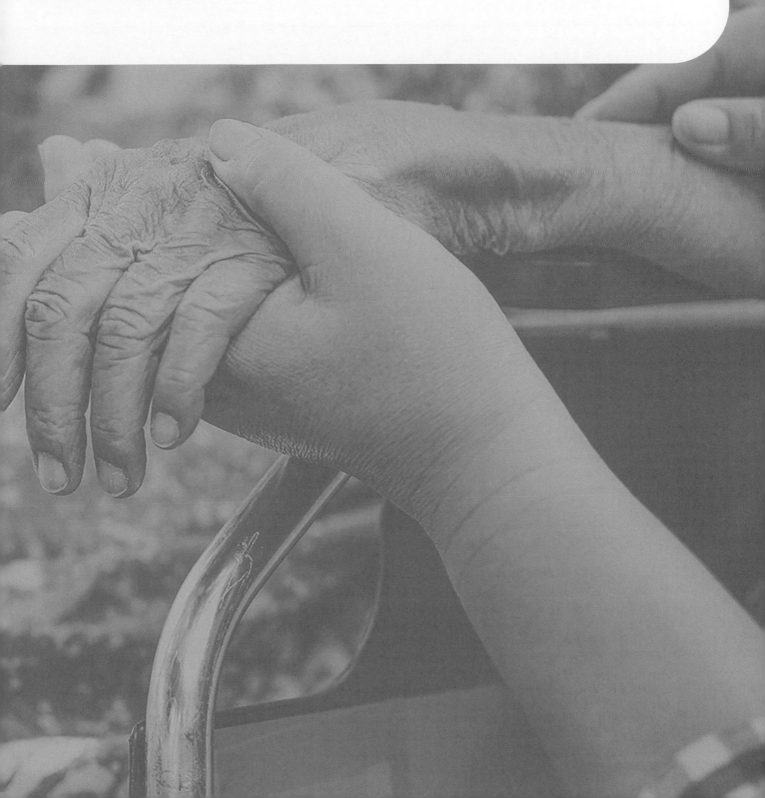

1. STRUCTURE AND PROFILE OF THE AGED CARE SECTOR

The Australian government collects taxes and funds the aged care sector. The aged care system focuses on two main forms of support delivery: residential care, and home and community support. Name three services that are delivered to care recipients in each of these support settings.

(pages 3–4 of Scott, Webb and Kostelnick, 5th edition)

Residential care:

_____

_____

_____

_____

_____

Home and community support:

_____

_____

_____

_____

_____

2. BEST PRACTICE SERVICE DELIVERY MODEL

(pages 4–6 of Scott, Webb and Kostelnick, 5th edition)

What is the main piece of legislation governing aged care facilities in Australia?

_____

_____

_____

In determining the standard of support provided to older people, the facility must fulfil a number of requirements. Name three of these.

_____

_____

_____

_____

What is the 'tool' used to determine care recipients' need for support under the *Aged Care Act 1997*?

_____

_____

_____

3. AGED CARE FACILITIES

(pages 6–9 of Scott, Webb and Kostelnick, 5th edition)

The purpose of an aged care facility is to provide a home-like environment and to promote physical and mental health matched to the individual needs of the care recipients. Name three goals of aged care facilities.

_____

_____

_____

The Role of the Support Worker

(pages 9–10 of Scott, Webb and Kostelnick, 5th edition)

Read Box 1.1 on page 11.

Personal Support Worker – Job Description

Read Table 1.2 on page 12.

Explain why it is important that you recognise your own limitations and work within your job role boundary (scope of practice).

What document might you refer to for guidance in understanding your role and role boundaries?

_____

_____

_____

_____

Identify some of the consequences that might arise if you do not follow instructions.

_____

_____

_____

_____

Identify some of the consequences that might arise if you were to perform work outside of your job role and boundaries.

_____

_____

_____

_____

Activity 1

In what circumstances could an aged care worker administer medications to a client?

_____

_____

_____

What would you do if a client requests you to do some personal shopping for them?

_____

_____

_____

4. OTHER SERVICES: THE MULTIDISCIPLINARY TEAM

(page 9 of Scott, Webb and Kostelnick, 5th edition)

To meet the many and varied support needs of care recipients, a network of agencies may be required. Name three organisations/healthcare professionals to whom the care recipient may be referred.

_____

_____

_____

Read Table 1.1. on page 9.

5. DUTY OF CARE

(page 16 of Scott, Webb and Kostelnick, 5th edition)

As a support worker, you have a duty of care to care recipients. What do you understand by 'duty of care'?

_____

_____

_____

_____

_____

In your workplace, how do you determine what is 'reasonable care' – that is, what is expected of you as a support worker?

_____

_____

_____

_____

_____

Activity 2

You take Mrs Black to the shower. She is frail and confused. While you are attending to Mrs Black in the shower, Mr Bloomfield calls out that he is going to be sick. You rush off to get Mr Bloomfield a vomit bowl. When you return, Mrs Black has fallen on the bathroom floor and hit her head.

Have you breached your duty of care? Give examples. How else could/should you have handled this situation?

_____

_____

_____

6. INFORMED CONSENT

(page 83 and 86 of Scott, Webb and Kostelnick, 5th edition)

For consent to be valid, the following criteria exist:

- The person must have the legal capacity.
- Consent must be given freely.
- Consent must be specific – that is, it relates only to the treatment or procedure about which the care recipient has been informed and has agreed to.
- Who can give informed consent?

_____

_____

_____

_____

_____

Activity 3

You are visiting one of your care recipients, Mr Jones, at his home. Mr Jones is of sound mind. He is complaining of chest pain and you are concerned that he might be having a heart attack. You ask Mr Jones if you can call an ambulance, but he refuses to go to hospital by ambulance.

Does Mr Jones have the right to withhold consent?

_____

_____

_____

_____

What should you do now?

_____

_____

_____

_____

7. ATTITUDES TO AGEING

(pages 156 of Scott, Webb and Kostelnick, 5th edition)

Attitudes to ageing vary across cultures. Many cultures view older people with respect, whereas in others a higher value is placed on youth.

Activity 4

Break into small groups. List three attitudes various cultures have when it comes to caring for the elderly. Once you have made your list, the trainer will ask you to present to the class for discussion.

_____

_____

_____

What do you understand by the term 'ageism'? Discuss this with your group.

_____

_____

_____

Activity 5: Ageism

Imagine that you are 87 years old. You take a little longer to do things than when you were younger, but you still live independently, do your own shopping, and do most of your housework and gardening.

How do you feel about being 87?

_____

_____

_____

How do you think the teenagers you see in the supermarket feel about you?

_____

_____

_____

What do you think the other drivers on the road think about you?

_____

_____

_____

What do you wish you were still able to do?

_____

_____

_____

8. ATTITUDES AND STEREOTYPES

The way people view others may be affected by their preconceived views or attitudes (stereotypes). As a support worker you must be aware of any stereotypical views you hold and work hard not to judge your care recipients by these views.

How would you describe a stereotype?

_____

_____

_____

Activity 6

Answer _True_ or _False_ for these statements, and then discuss your views with your group.

All old people get dementia.	True/False
All young people don't want a job.	True/False
Older people cannot learn new things.	True/False
Most people aged over 75 live in nursing homes.	True/False

9. SOCIAL DEVALUATION

Social devaluation is negative social judgement based on some characteristic of a person or group. This may lead to a person feeling rejected by others, or having a sense of worthlessness, despair, loss of control, freedom and insecurity. Some care recipients in aged care facilities may be in danger of suffering from social devaluation. In discussion with your group and trainer, list three strategies you could implement to prevent a care recipient from suffering from social devaluation.

_____

_____

_____

_____

_____

10. COMMON CHALLENGES ASSOCIATED WITH AGEING

The main challenge with ageing relates to maintaining quality health. Older people are a source of skills and experience that can greatly benefit society. To realise this benefit, an older person needs to be supported by a healthy social and physical environment.

Name three main challenges an older person faces.

_____

_____

_____

_____

What makes for quality ageing? Identify three main points.

_____

_____

_____

_____

11. HEALTH NEEDS

(page 123 of Scott, Webb and Kostelnick, 5th edition)

Read Box 5.4 on page 123.

One of many personal tasks that a person needs assistance with is the management of their health needs. Health needs include:

_____

_____

12. THE NURSING PROCESS

(pages 102–105 of Scott, Webb and Kostelnick, 5th edition)

The nursing process is used to identify and plan support for a person. As a support worker, you might be asked to collect information that is then used to create the plan of support. The nursing process is also used to assess a person. The nursing process has five steps:

1 _____

_____

_____

_____

2 _____

_____

_____

_____

3 _____

_____

_____

_____

_____

4 _____
_____
_____
_____
_____

5 _____
_____
_____
_____
_____

Who should be involved in the development of a person-centred plan?

_____
_____
_____

Identify the support services that might be relevant to successfully implement the person-centred plan.

_____
_____
_____

13. OBSERVATIONS

It is important that you have the ability to identify signs and symptoms that indicate a change in a person's condition. You must be aware of signs that suggest a person's situation may be adversely changing.

What is the difference between objective data and subjective data?

_____
_____
_____
_____

Take some time to read through Box 4.1, 'Basic observations' on page 102 of Scott, Webb and Kostelnick, 5th edition and complete the activity below.

Activity 7

Next to each disorder in the table below, list at least two signs and two symptoms for each disorder that the person might experience.

Disorder	Sign	Symptom
Heart failure		
Dementia		
Asthma		
Gum disease		
Urinary tract infection		

Physical Perspective

Complete the table using the Nursing Process method.

Risk/Situation	Assessment	Goals	Strategy	Documentation and Evaluation
Kevin is incontinent and is developing a rash in his groin.				
Kevin is no longer able to dress himself and tie his own shoelaces.				
Kevin is not eating.				
Kevin likes to sleep all day, but cannot sleep at night.				

14. PERSON-CENTRED SUPPORT

(pages 21 of Scott, Webb and Kostelnick, 5th edition)

The person-centred care approach is based around placing the aged person at the centre of the care. The focus is on the individual requiring the care. It involves assessing needs and planning care to meet those individual needs.

Activity 8

Answer *Yes* or *No* for these statements as examples of person-centred support:

Refer to women as 'sweetie' and men as 'old codger'.	Yes/No
Let the aged person be the judge of what is in their best interest.	Yes/No
Ask the aged person how they would like something done.	Yes/No
Use respectful listening and communicating skills.	Yes/No

15. ELDER ABUSE

(pages 87–89 of Scott, Webb and Kostelnick, 5th edition)

Read Box 3.1 on page 88.

Elder abuse is a pattern of behaviour that causes physical, psychological, financial or social harm to an older person, including as a result of neglect. Abuse may be carried out by partners, friends, family members, carers or health professionals. Abuse can occur at home or in a residential aged care setting.

Support workers owe a duty of care to care recipients to keep them safe. People with dementia are more likely to be abused, as they cannot always speak up about the abuse and so it may go undetected.

Activity 9

For each type of abuse, list some indications for that abuse.

Type of abuse	Indications of abuse
Physical	
Psychological	
Financial	
Sexual	
Neglect	

Activity 10

You are working in an aged care facility or community environment. You observe that one of the support workers seems to have a dislike for a male care recipient. The care recipient needs more attention than other care recipients, which appears to irritate the support worker.

When meals are being served and the particular support worker is on the shift bringing the meals to care recipients' rooms, you notice that the male care recipient is always the last person to receive their meal and it is cold.

Do you consider this to be a form of abuse?

_____

_____

_____

If you consider this to be a form of abuse, what type would you classify it as?

_____

_____

_____

What does Australian legislation state about reporting elder abuse?

_____

_____

_____

What steps must you take according to your employer's policies and procedures?

_____

_____

_____

_____

Why might abuse or neglect not be reported?

_____

_____

_____

_____

16. RESTRICTIVE PRACTICES

(pages 85–86 of Scott, Webb and Kostelnick, 5th edition)

What is meant by a 'restraint-free environment'?

_____

_____

_____

In what circumstances can restraints be used?

_____

_____

_____

Name the different types of restraints that can be used and give an example of each.

_____

_____

_____

_____

What factors would you consider in using a restrictive practice?

_____

_____

_____

17. MONITORING RESTRICTIVE PRACTICES

A registered nurse must maintain the restraint records. What should be included in the restraint record?

_____

_____

_____

18. HUMAN RIGHTS

(page 90 of Scott, Webb and Kostelnick, 5th edition)

Read Box 3.2 Charter of Care Recipients' Rights and Responsibilities

Activity 11

Mrs Williams is 90 years old. She does not have any cognitive impairment. However, she has become increasingly frail and is at risk of falls. Mrs Williams walks with a walking frame.

Mrs Williams wants to walk to the toilet and the dining room unaided. Her family members are worried that she might fall and don't want her walking anymore.

What are Mrs Williams's rights?

_____

_____

_____

What strategies could you implement to make it safer for Mrs Williams to walk to the toilet and dining room?

_____

_____

_____

_____

19. CARE RECIPIENTS' RIGHTS TO MAKE PERSONAL CHOICES

(pages 92 of Scott, Webb and Kostelnick, 5th edition)

What personal choices can care recipients make?

_____

_____

_____

_____

20. THE MEDICAL RECORD

(pages 99–102 of Scott, Webb and Kostelnick, 5th edition)

The medical record is organised into sections.

Activity 12

Give an example of what information must be written in each section.

Admission sheet	
Medical history	
Physical examination results	
Doctors' orders	
Progress notes	
Aged care assessment team (ACAT) report	
Observation sheets	
Social history	
Pathology results	
Alternative therapies notes	
Special consents	

21. REPORTING AND RECORDING

(pages 105–106 of Scott, Webb and Kostelnick, 5th edition)

Read Box 4.2 on page 106, Rules for Recording/Reporting.

Reporting means giving an oral account of support and observations.

Recording means writing an account of observations and support. It is often called report writing or documenting.

You must report every change that affects a care recipient's needs. You should not wait until someone else notices the change or leave it to someone else to report it.

List 10 changes you might notice in your care recipient that would require you to provide an oral report immediately and subsequently require you to document.

1. _____
2. _____
3. _____
4. _____
5. _____
6. _____
7. _____
8. _____
9. _____
10. _____

Reporting

When reporting, follow these rules:

_____

_____

_____

_____

_____

_____

_____

End-of-Shift Report

The end-of-shift report is also known as the handover. What are some important points you need to note about the handover report?

_____

_____

_____

_____

Check whether your organisation requires you to record time in conventional time or by using the 24-hour clock.

Read Box 4.2 on pages 106 and discuss with your trainer.

Activity 13

Progress Notes

You have been caring for an 88-year-old care recipient, Mr Lightfoot, at your facility. Mr Lightfoot has been assigned to you from 7.00 a.m. to 3.00 p.m. (0700 to 1500). When you took him to the shower, you noticed an ulcer developing on his right ankle. It looks very red and the skin is starting to break. Mr Lightfoot is a diabetic. He didn't eat very much of his breakfast today – only half a Weet-Bix and a cup of tea. You take his blood sugar level (BSL) – also referred to as blood glucose level (BGL) – and the reading is 2.1. You also notice that he is confused. He is normally very lucid and likes to talk. You have other care recipients to care for. Progress notes are usually written at the end of the day.

Should you wait until 3.00 p.m. (1500) to write Mr Lightfoot's progress notes? What should you do immediately?

_____

_____

_____

_____

_____

_____

Write your report on Mr Lightfoot in the table below.

Surname: Lightfoot	
Given Name: Gordon	
DOB: 12/12/1927	
Waterfall Aged Care Facility	
PROGRESS NOTES	
Date/Time	**Comments**

22. PRIVACY AND CONFIDENTIALITY

(page 92 of Scott, Webb and Kostelnick, 5th edition)

Care recipients have a right to personal privacy.

List all the things you can think of that relate to a care recipient's personal privacy.

_____

_____

_____

How can you maintain a care recipient's confidentiality?

_____

_____

_____

How does your facility/community organisation ensure that care recipients' information is stored securely and confidentiality is maintained? You may currently work in a facility. If you do not, you will find this information when you attend your work placement.

_____

_____

_____

_____

23. USE OF DIGITAL TECHNOLOGY

(pages 110–111 of Scott, Webb and Kostelnick, 5th edition)

Read Box 4.3 on p. 111 and discuss with your trainer and the group.

What are some advantages of a computer management system?

_____

_____

_____

_____

_____

24. PREVENTING FALLS

What factors increase the risk of a fall?

_____

_____

_____

What safety measures could you put into place to prevent falls?

_____

_____

_____

_____

_____

25. RISK MANAGEMENT

(pages 42–45 of Scott, Webb and Kostelnick, 5th edition)

Risk is defined as the possibility an event (incident or occurrence) will occur and adversely affect the achievement of objectives.

Risk management is the practice of systematically identifying and assessing, mitigating (reducing), monitoring and reporting risks and the controls that are in place to manage and treat them.

The four steps involved in the risk management process are:

Step 1 – Identify the risk

Step 2 – Assess the risk

Step 3 – Treat/control the risk

Step 4 – Monitor effectiveness of treatment/control

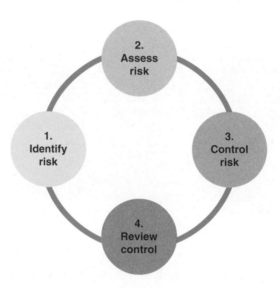

Figure 1.1 Risk management process.

What is a risk?

_____

_____

_____

What are the four steps in the risk management process?

_____

_____

_____

How do you report risks, accidents and incidents at your workplace?

_____

_____

Identifying Risks

Workplace risks can be identified by workplace inspection, checking injury records, consulting workers and looking at workers' compensation statistics.

Once you have identified a workplace risk, you need to assess the level of risk. A risk matrix is a table that is used during risk assessment to define the level of risk by considering the category of likelihood of the adverse event or incident occurring against the category of consequence or impact of the adverse event or incident. The comparison of a level of impact with likelihood will enable a level of risk severity to be determined.

An example of a risk matrix is provided below.

When undertaking a risk assessment you need to firstly assess the consequence or impact of the adverse event or incident <u>before</u> you assess the likelihood of the adverse event or incident occurring.

Once the risk has been assessed, we need to implement control measures to reduce the likelihood of the adverse event occurring.

The hierarchy of control is a series of steps that should be followed to eliminate or reduce risk. The steps are listed from most effective to least effective (see Fig. 1.3).

Activity 14

How are risks identified at your workplace?

_____

_____

Break up into groups of two or three people. Using the table on the last page of this workbook, write down one risk you can think of in your workplace. Assess the level of risk using the risk assessment matrix below and then work out what control measures would be suitable to eliminate or minimise the risk. Refer to the hierarchy of controls diagram (Fig. 1.3) when working out your control measures. Record the results in the table.

Likelihood of harm	Consequence of harm		
	Major Death, major injury/illness, long-term disability	**Moderate** Moderate injury/illness requiring treatment at a hospital, short-term disability	**Minor** Minor injury/illness requiring treatment at the workplace, no disability
Probable (highly likely to occur more than once in the next 12 months)	High	High	Medium
Possible (likely to occur once in the next 24 months)	High	Medium	Low
Improbable (unlikely to occur once in the next 5 years)	Medium	Low	Low

Figure 1.2 Risk assessment matrix.

Assess risks – Develop assessment criteria – Likelihood/Frequency

- Likelihood represents the number of times within a specified period in which an event or action (risk) may occur and the assessed probability of occurrence of the event or action.
- Likelihood grading levels can be expressed as frequency of occurrence:
  - **Probable** (Highly Likely to occur more than once in the next 12 months)
  - **Possible** (Likely to occur once in the next 24 months)
  - **Improbable** (Unlikely to occur once in the next 5 years)
- An important aspect to consider when estimating likelihood is the frequency and duration of exposure of employees to the risk. This can range from infrequent to continuous. Frequency of exposure is the proportion of an employee's working hours during which they are exposed to a particular risk/hazard.

Assess risks – Develop assessment criteria – Impact/Consequences

- Impact (or consequence) refers to the extent to which the occurrence of a risk event might harm an individual. Extent of harm to the individual (worker or care recipient) grading levels can be expressed as:
  - **Major** (death, major injury or illness normally resulting in long term disability).
  - **Moderate** (moderate injury or illness requiring treatment at a hospital normally resulting in short term disability).
  - **Minor** (minor injury or illness requiring treatment at the workplace with no resultant disability).

Assess risks – Develop assessment criteria – Risk Severity

- Risk severity is the risk rating derived from the aggregation of the assessed likelihood and the **highest impact** on a risk heat map. The risk severity band should be viewed from a residual risk perspective to reflect the current status of a risk (i.e. controls exist to manage inherent risks, therefore they should be considered in the overall assessment of the risk profile).
- The risk severity ratings used are based on a three-tier grading level for the **Likelihood** and **Consequence** of an identified risk (such as Norovirus outbreak) happening. The scale used to rate each overall risk is the product (combination) of **Consequence and Likelihood** and is assessed as follows:
  - High
  - Medium
  - Low

Hierarchy of Control

CONTROL MEASURES

Use the right controls to eliminate or minimise risks and to protect your workers.

ELIMINATION

Remove the hazard completely.
Eliminating the hazard is the most effective way to manage risks.

Where it is not practical to eliminate a hazard,
risk must be minimised.

Use one or more of the following:

Engineering	Substitute the hazard	Isolate the hazard
Change the design	Replace the hazard with	Separate the hazard from people

Minimise any remaining risk by using
administrative controls.

ADMINISTRATION

Health and safety procedures and policies,
e.g. safe work procedures, staff training.

If risks remain, the possible impact on people
must be controlled using PPE.

PERSONAL PROTECTIVE EQUIPMENT (PPE)

e.g. safety glasses, hard hats, protective clothing.
This is the least effective way to manage risks.

To find out more, visit **safework.nsw.gov.au** or call us on **13 10 50.**

SW09182 0219   SAFEWORK NSW

Figure 1.3 Hierarchy of control.
(SafeWork, NSW Government, Australia. Available at: www.safework.nsw.gov.au/__data/assets/pdf_file/0006/446028/hierarchy-of-controls-SW09182.pdf)

The **Hierarchy of control** is a series of steps that should be followed to eliminate or reduce risk. The steps are listed from most effective to least effective.

1 **Elimination** – get rid of the hazard altogether, e.g. manually lifting residents must be eliminated

2 **Substitution** – replace the hazardous practice with a less hazardous one, e.g. use a mechanical lifter, or if soap is giving support workers dermatitis, substitute the soap with a hypoallergenic handwash

3 **Engineering** – ventilation system, height adjustable bed, wheels on trolley and chairs.

4 **Isolation** – store room for chemicals and locked cupboard for S8 drugs, sound-proofing

5 **Administrative** controls, such as policies and procedures, job rotation, training, redesigning jobs

6 **Personal Protective Equipment** (PPE) is always last resort, as you should explore all the options above first. Also human nature dictates that people don't always wear their PPE. Examples, earmuffs, eye protection, masks and gloves.

Risk	Risk Severity Rating			Control Measures (What steps will we take to reduce the risk severity rating?)	Monitoring and Supervision (How will the compliance with the control measures be supervised and monitored?)	Person Responsible
	Likelihood	Consequence	Severity			
Failure to follow hand hygiene procedures (which can lead to spread of infection)	Probable	Major	High	**Administrative:** Policies, procedures, infection control manual. Education and training. Provision of hand hygiene products – allocate responsibility in statement of duties Electronic reporting system	Monthly hand hygiene audits. Appoint infection control coordinator. Training records Competency assessment	Infection Control Coordinator Registered Nurse Educator All support staff

2

Unit HLTWHS002:
Follow safe work practices for direct client care

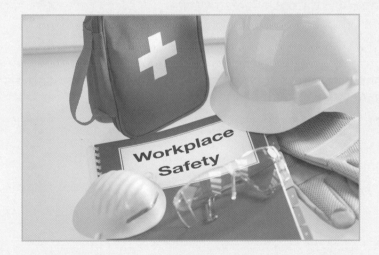

Figure 2.1 Workplace health and safety
(iStockphoto/YinYang)

Table of Contents

INTRODUCTION

This workbook relates to the unit **HLTWHS002: Follow safe work practices for direct client care**.

The workbook activities and final assessment tasks will enable you to:

- follow safe work practices for direct client care
- follow safe work practices for manual handling
- follow safe work practices for infection control
- contribute to safe work practices in the workplace
- reflect on your own safe work practices.

To prepare for this unit and the assessment activities, we recommend that you first read Chapter 2 of Scott, Webb and Kostelnick, 5th edition, **Protecting the person and the carer**.

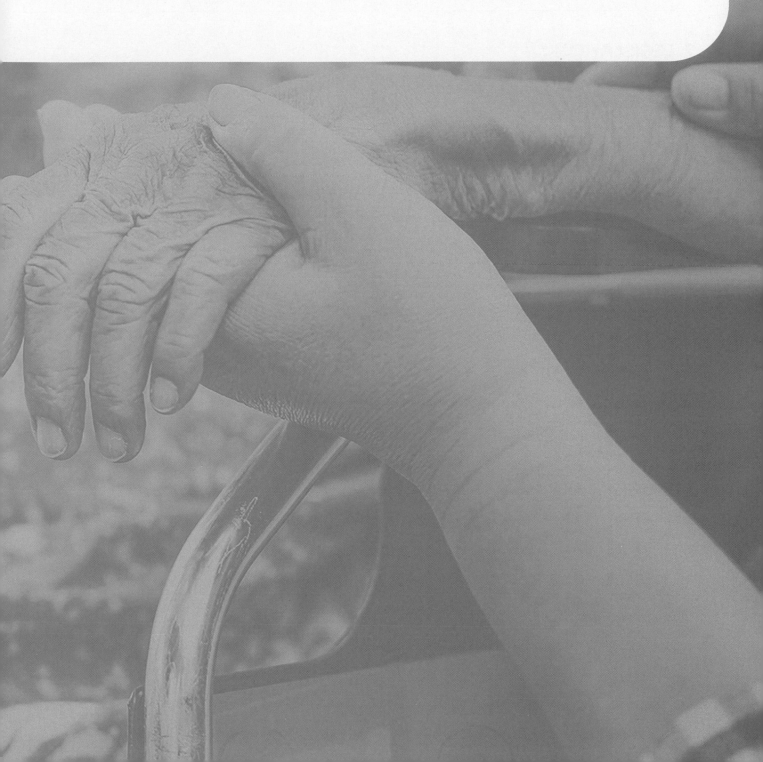

1. SAFETY

(page 26 of Scott, Webb and Kostelnick, 5th edition)

How would you describe a safe work environment?

_____

_____

_____

What factors increase the client's risk of accident or injury?

_____

_____

_____

2. LEGISLATION

(page 26 of Scott, Webb and Kostelnick, 5th edition)

What is the name of the legislation that covers all workplaces in Australia?

_____

_____

_____

_____

_____

3. DUE DILIGENCE

Officers have a duty to exercise 'due diligence' to ensure the person conducting a business or undertaking (PCBU) complies with its duties under the _Work Health and Safety Act 2011_. They are to take reasonable steps to:

_____

_____

_____

_____

4. 'REASONABLY PRACTICABLE'

'Reasonably practicable', as defined under section 18 of the Work, Health and Safety Act, states that there is a requirement to weigh up all matters, including:

_____

_____

_____

_____

5. HOME HAZARD ASSESSMENT

(page 27 of Scott, Webb and Kostelnick, 5th edition)

Activity 1

Read through Box 2.1 on page 27. Think of a client's home or your own home, and spend 15 minutes or so discussing with your trainer the areas of your client's home or your own home that do not comply with safety in the home.

What about pets? What risk can they present to the client or carer?

After having read the box, write down at least five things you could improve in your own home or a client's home you have visited recently.

1. _____
2. _____
3. _____
4. _____
5. _____

6. PREVENTING FALLS

(pages 28–31 of Scott, Webb and Kostelnick, 5th edition)

What factors increase the risk of a fall?

_____
_____
_____

What safety measures could you put into place to prevent falls?

_____
_____
_____
_____
_____
_____

7. PREVENTING POISONING

(pages 31–32 of Scott, Webb and Kostelnick, 5th edition)

Accidental poisoning in an aged care facility and in the home is a health hazard. How could you prevent accidental poisoning?

_____
_____
_____
_____
_____

8. PREVENTING BURNS

(pages 32–33 of Scott, Webb and Kostelnick, 5th edition)

Burns are a leading cause of death, especially among children and older people. What safety measures could be put into place to prevent burns?

_____

_____

_____

_____

_____

_____

9. PREVENTING SUFFOCATION

(page 33 of Scott, Webb and Kostelnick, 5th edition)

Suffocation is when breathing stops from lack of oxygen. The following safety measures can help prevent suffocation:

_____

_____

_____

_____

_____

_____

10. PREVENTING EQUIPMENT-RELATED ACCIDENTS

(pages 33–34 of Scott, Webb and Kostelnick, 5th edition)

Equipment must be kept in safe working order. How do you do this?

_____

_____

_____

_____

_____

_____

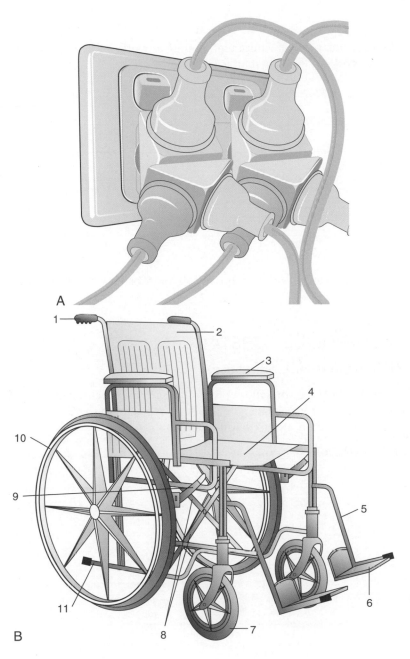

1. Handgrip/push handle
2. Back upholstery
3. Armrest
4. Seat upholstery
5. Front rigging
6. Footplate
7. Caster
8. Crossbrace
9. Wheel lock
10. Wheel and handrim
11. Tipping lever

Figure 2.2 Preventing equipment-related accidents. **A.** An overloaded electrical outlet. **B.** Wheelchair safety

(A: Redrawn based on Sorrentino A & Gorek B, 2003, Mosby's Textbook for Long-Term Care Assistants, 4th edn, Mosby, St Louis.
B: Reproduced with permission from Sorrentino A & Gorek B, 2011, Mosby's Textbook for Long-Term Care Nursing Assistants, 6th edn, Mosby, St Louis.)

Activity 2

Break into small groups. Look at one piece of equipment you use at work, and write down how you would inspect the equipment and ensure it is working in a safe manner.

_____

_____

_____

_____

_____

_____

Take some time to read Box 2.5 on page 34 of the Scott, Webb and Kostelnick, 5th edition, and discuss it with your trainer and the rest of the group.

11. HANDLING HAZARDOUS SUBSTANCES

(pages 34–37 of Scott, Webb and Kostelnick, 5th edition)

A hazardous substance is any chemical that presents a physical hazard or a health hazard in the workplace. List below some hazardous substances used at your workplace, the results of exposure to these substances and safety measures taken to ensure that these substances do not cause harm to anyone.

Check your answers against Box 2.7 on page 36.

Hazardous substance	Safety measures to put into place when handling hazardous substances

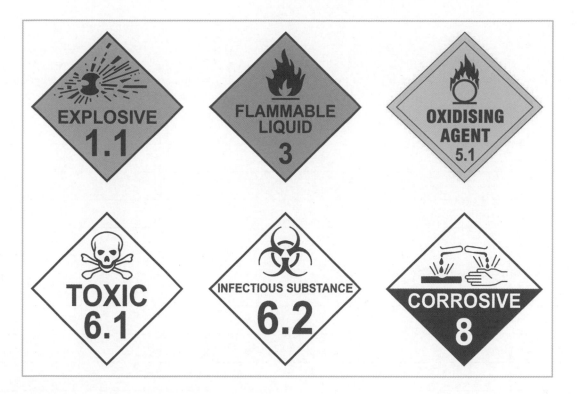

Figure 2.3 Warning labels on hazardous substances
(Reproduced with permission from Sorrentino A & Gorek B (2003). Mosby's textbook for long-term care assistants, 4th edn, Mosby, St Louis.)

12. SAFETY DATA SHEETS (SDS)

(page 37 of Scott, Webb and Kostelnick, 5th edition)

What is a Safety Data Sheet (SDS), and what does it tell you about the hazardous substance?

_____

_____

_____

_____

_____

_____

_____

13. FIRE SAFETY

(pages 37–38 of Scott, Webb and Kostelnick, 5th edition)

Are fire prevention methods in place in all aged care environments? Read Box 2.8 on page 37.

_____

_____

_____

_____

_____

_____

Activity 3

What to do if there is a fire

It is important to know your aged care facility's policies and procedures for fire emergencies. Know where to find fire alarms, fire extinguishers and emergency exits. Fire drills are held to practise emergency fire procedures. Remember the acronym RACE. What does it stand for?

R _____

A _____

C _____

E _____

What is the procedure for using a fire extinguisher?

1 _____

2 _____

3 _____

4 _____

5 _____

6 _____

7 _____

Your trainer will now **simulate** the procedure for using a fire extinguisher using an actual fire extinguisher from the workplace.

14. EVACUATION

(page 38 of Scott, Webb and Kostelnick, 5th edition)

Activity 4

What is the procedure for evacuating clients at your workplace?

_____

_____

_____

_____

_____

15. WORKPLACE VIOLENCE

(pages 39 of Scott, Webb and Kostelnick, 5th edition)

Violence can happen in the workplace, and the aged care facility is no exception. Although most health workplace-related violence occur in acute healthcare settings, it can still happen in an aged care facility.

List some factors associated with work-related assaults in aged care facilities, and suggest control measures that could be put into place to prevent these incidents.

Work-related violence incident	Control measures

Read Boxes 2.9 and 2.10 on page 41. Your trainer will discuss with you these practices for preventing violence and ensuring personal safety.

16. RISK MANAGEMENT

(page 42 of Scott, Webb and Kostelnick, 5th edition)

Risk management involves identifying and controlling risk and safety hazards that affect the aged care facility.

What is a risk?

_____

_____

_____

What is the difference between an accident and an incident?

_____

_____

_____

How do you report hazards, accidents and incidents at your workplace?

_____

_____

_____

Identifying Risks

Workplace hazards can be identified by workplace inspection, checking injury records, consulting workers and looking at workers' compensation statistics.

How are hazards identified at your workplace?

_____

_____

_____

_____

Once you have identified a hazard, you need to assess the level of risk. This means the likelihood of injury or illness, and the severity of the injury or illness that results from exposure to the hazard.

An example of a risk matrix is given in Fig. 1.2 (see p. 21). Once the risk has been assessed, we need to implement control measures (refer to Fig. 1.3, p. 23).

Activity 5

Break up into groups of two or three people. Write down one hazard you can think of in your workplace. Assess the level of risk using the risk assessment matrix in your Practical Assessment and then work out what control measures would be suitable to eliminate or minimise the risk. Refer to the hierarchy of controls in your Practical Assessment when working out your control measures.

_____

_____

_____

_____

_____

One person from each group will present their risk assessment and control measures to the class. The trainer will write answers on the whiteboard and then brainstorm the rest of the class for any additional control measures they would like to add.

17. MANUAL HANDLING AND BODY MECHANICS

(pages 45–47 of Scott, Webb and Kostelnick, 5th edition)

'A hazardous manual task means a task that requires a person to lift, lower, push, pull, carry or otherwise move, hold or restrain any person, animal or thing involving one of more of the following:

- repetitive or sustained force
- high or sudden force
- repetitive movement
- sustained or awkward posture
- exposure to vibration.'

(SafeWork NSW – www.safework.nsw.gov.au)

To work safely you must be familiar with the Hazardous Manual Tasks Code of Practice. What does this code of practice cover in relation to hazardous manual tasks?

_____

_____

_____

_____

We often talk about _good posture_, _base of support_ and _body mechanics_. What do we mean by these terms?

_____

_____

_____

_____

_____

'An injury sustained while carrying out a hazardous manual task is called a musculoskeletal disorder (MSD). MSDs occur due to:

1. Wear and tear to joints, ligaments, muscles and inter-vertebral discs caused by repeated or continuous use of the same body parts, including static body positions.

2. Sudden damage caused by strenuous activity, or unexpected movements such as when loads being handled move or change position suddenly.'

(SafeWork NSW, www.workcover.nsw.gov.au)

Name some common MSDs caused through performing hazardous manual tasks.

_____

_____

_____

_____

_____

_____

18. BACK CARE

(pages 47–48 of Scott, Webb and Kostelnick, 5th edition)

Read the Safety Alert on page 47.

What are common signs and symptoms for someone who has a back injury?

_____

_____

_____

_____

How do we maintain a healthy spine?

_____

_____

_____

_____

List at least five rules for correct manual handling techniques (see page 47).

_____

_____

_____

_____

_____

_____

Activity 6

Perform the following practical exercises, either in the workplace or in a simulated workplace environment.

The exercises can be found in the Final Assessment section of this workbook. You will practise these exercises with your trainer before being assessed at the workplace.

- Moving a client in bed
- Raising the client's head and shoulders
- Log rolling
- Transferring a client from bed to chair
- Transferring a client using a walk belt
- Transferring a client using a mechanical lifter and stand up lifter
- Moving a client in bed using a slide sheet
- Assisting a client from a wheelchair into a car

19. INFECTION PREVENTION AND CONTROL

(pages 68–75 of Scott, Webb and Kostelnick, 5th edition)

What is the difference between pathogens and normal flora?

_____

_____

_____

_____

What are the four types of microorganisms?

_____

_____

_____

_____

20. INFECTION

(pages 68–70 of Scott, Webb and Kostelnick, 5th edition)

An infection is a disease state resulting from the invasion and growth of microorganisms in the body. A local infection is in a body part – for example, conjunctivitis is an infection of the eye. A systemic infection involves the whole body – examples are septicaemia and measles. Signs and symptoms of infection include:

_____

_____

_____

_____

Why are older people who live in residential aged care more susceptible to infection?

Write your answers below, and then compare them with Box 2.15 on page 68.

_____

_____

_____

_____

What is meant by 'Standard Precautions'?

_____

_____

_____

_____

Additional Precautions

Additional precautions such as isolation, personal protective equipment (PPE) and disposable crockery and cutlery are applied when a client has a highly contagious disease such as measles, chicken pox or methicillin-resistant *Staphylococcus aureus*.

A common infection in residential facilities is gastroenteritis. The Department of Social Services (previously the Department of Health and Ageing) has published an Outbreak Coordinators Handbook to assist staff of residential aged care facilities in the event of a gastroenteritis outbreak.

The Outbreak Management Kit can be downloaded from the Department of Social Services website. It includes all the information needed to manage a gastroenteritis outbreak, including an:

- outbreak management checklist
- outbreak flow chart
- outbreak management plan
- outbreak management plan template.

Download and read a copy of the kit to prepare for your final assessment.

Chain of infection

_____

_____

_____

_____

_____

_____

21. HAND HYGIENE

(pages 71–73 of Scott, Webb and Kostelnick, 5th edition)

Why are handwashing and hand hygiene so important when working in residential aged care, hospitals and in the community with clients?

_____

_____

_____

_____

_____

_____

When do you need to wash your hands?

_____

_____

_____

_____

Read the rules of handwashing on page 72.

Activity 7

Practical exercises on hand hygiene can be found in the Final Assessment section of this workbook. You will practise these exercises with your trainer before being assessed at the workplace or in a simulated workplace environment.

Your Moments for
Hand Hygiene
Health care in a residential home

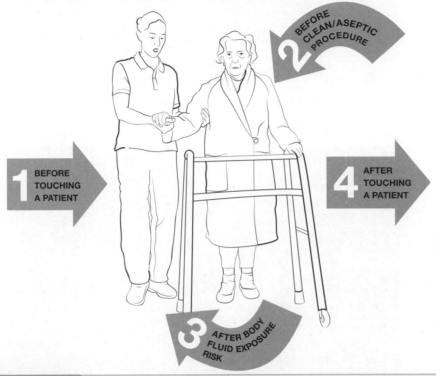

1	BEFORE TOUCHING A PATIENT	WHEN?	Clean your hands before touching a patient.
		WHY?	To protect the patient against harmful germs carried on your hands.
2	BEFORE CLEAN/ ASEPTIC PROCEDURE	WHEN?	Clean your hands immediately before performing a clean/aseptic procedure.
		WHY?	To protect the patient against harmful germs, including the patient's own, from entering his/her body.
3	AFTER BODY FLUID EXPOSURE RISK	WHEN?	Clean your hands immediately after a procedure involving exposure risk to body fluids (and after glove removal).
		WHY?	To protect yourself and the environment from harmful patient germs.
4	AFTER TOUCHING A PATIENT	WHEN?	Clean your hands after touching the patient at the end of the encounter or when the encounter is interrupted.
		WHY?	To protect yourself and the environment from harmful patient germs.

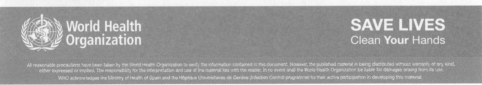

World Health Organization

SAVE LIVES
Clean **Your** Hands

All reasonable precautions have been taken by the World Health Organization to verify the information contained in this document. However, the published material is being distributed without warranty of any kind, either expressed or implied. The responsibility for the interpretation and use of the material lies with the reader. In no event shall the World Health Organization be liable for damages arising from its use.
WHO acknowledges the Ministry of Health of Spain and the Hôpitaux Universitaires de Genève (Infection Control programme) for their active participation in developing this material.

March 2012

Figure 2.4 Your moments for hand hygiene
(Reprinted from World Health Organisation, Your Moments for Hand Hygiene Health Care in a Residential Home Poster, www.who.int/gpsc/5may/residential-care.pdf.)

Personal protective equipment

(pages 73–75 of Scott, Webb and Kostelnick, 5th edition)

When should the following personal protective equipment (PPE) be worn?

Gloves	
Mask	
Eye protection (goggles)	
Apron or gown	

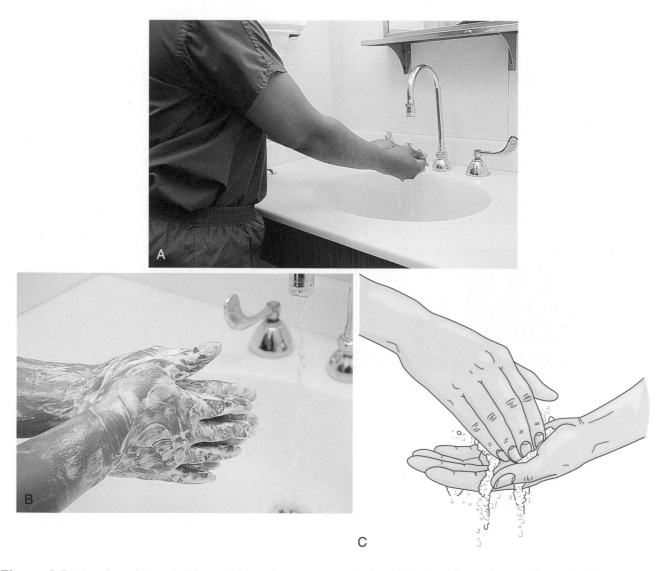

Figure 2.5 Handwashing. **A**. The uniform does not touch the sink. Hands are lower than the elbows. **B**. The palms are rubbed together for a good lather. **C**. Fingertips are rubbed against the palms to clean underneath the nails.

(Sorrentino A & Gorek B, 2010, Mosby's Textbook for Long-Term Care Assistants, Mosby, St Louis.)

22. ENVIRONMENTAL CONTROL AND CONTAMINATED WASTE

(page 76 of Scott, Webb and Kostelnick, 5th edition)

Good housekeeping, hygienic care and handling of laundry and correct disposal of waste are all essential elements of infection control. Waste should be segregated at the point of generation. Most healthcare and aged care facilities use appropriately colour-coded and labelled containers.

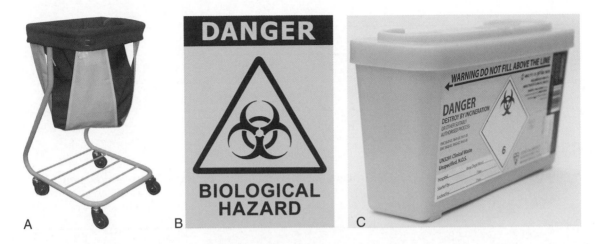

Figure 2.6 Clinical waste including linen skips, biological hazard signs and sharps containers
(Dalcross Medical Equipment (Linen skip); iStockphoto/Brilt (BioHazard sign); iStockphoto/DavidFR (sharps container))

Name an example of each of the following types of waste, and state in which coloured container you would place it.

Waste	Example	Container
Infectious or clinical waste		
Sharps		
Chemical-related waste		
Cytotoxic waste		
General waste		

23. SPILLS MANAGEMENT

(page 76 of Scott, Webb and Kostelnick, 5th edition)

Standard Precautions apply in the management of spills. What is the procedure for a spill of blood or body fluids?

_____

_____

_____

_____

24. LINEN AND LAUNDRY SERVICES

(page 76 of Scott, Webb and Kostelnick, 5th edition)

Aged care facilities and organisations have documented policies regarding procedures for the collection, transport, processing and storage of linen.

What is the procedure at your facility?

_____

_____

_____

_____

25. PERSONAL HEALTH

It is also important for staff working in the healthcare setting to maintain personal health and hygiene. How do staff do this?

_____

_____

_____

_____

26. FOCUSING ON COMMUNITY CARE

List four risks relating to caring for someone in their own home, and the control measures that could be put into place for each risk (remember the hierarchy of controls):

Hazard	Control measure
1	
2	
3	
4	

27. CONTRIBUTING TO SAFE WORK PRACTICES IN THE WORKPLACE

Activity 8

Who are the members of your Work Health and Safety Committee?

_____

_____

_____

_____

Case scenario

You are working the afternoon shift and notice that some of your work colleagues are not using the correct manual handling equipment. Instead, they are lifting the clients by themselves.

What risk does this practice pose to the staff member and the client? To whom should you report this matter? What do the policies and procedures at your workplace state with regards to manual handling?

_____

_____

_____

_____

28. REFLECTING ON YOUR OWN SAFE WORK PRACTICES

Activity 9

How can you maintain currency of safe work practices in relation to work health and safety, the use of equipment and infection control in your work role?

_____

_____

_____

_____

29. QUALITY OF LIFE

(page 79 of Scott, Webb and Kostelnick, 5th edition)

Activity 10

Read and discuss case study 1. Thinking back to the hierarchy of controls, with elimination being at the top of the list, do you think the risks have been eliminated or reduced? What if Margery decides not to go outside the lounge to smoke? What if she decides to have a bath, instead of a shower? If she is of sound mind, is she able to make these decisions to smoke inside the lounge and to have a bath? What about your health and safety when attending Margery's premises? What else could be done now to eliminate or reduce the risks?

_____

_____

_____

_____

_____

_____

_____

_____

Unit CHCLEG001:
Work legally and ethically

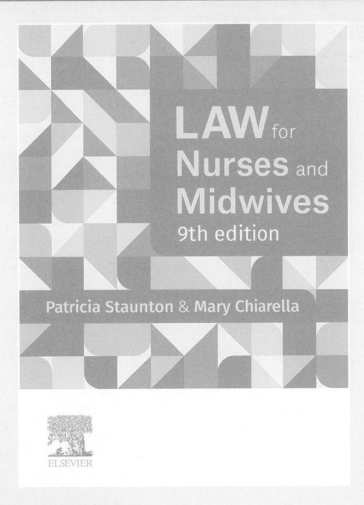

Figure 3.1 Law for Nurses and Midwives
(Staunton and Chiarella, 2020, Law for Nurses and Midwives, 9th ed, Elsevier, Australia.)

Table of Contents

INTRODUCTION

This workbook relates to the unit **CHCLEG001: Work legally and ethically**.

The workbook activities and final assessment tasks will enable you to:

- identify and respond to legal requirements
- identify and meet ethical responsibilities
- contribute to workplace improvements.

To prepare for this unit and the assessment activities, we recommend that you first read Chapter 3 of Scott, Webb and Kostelnick, 5th edition, **Working within a legal and ethical environment**.

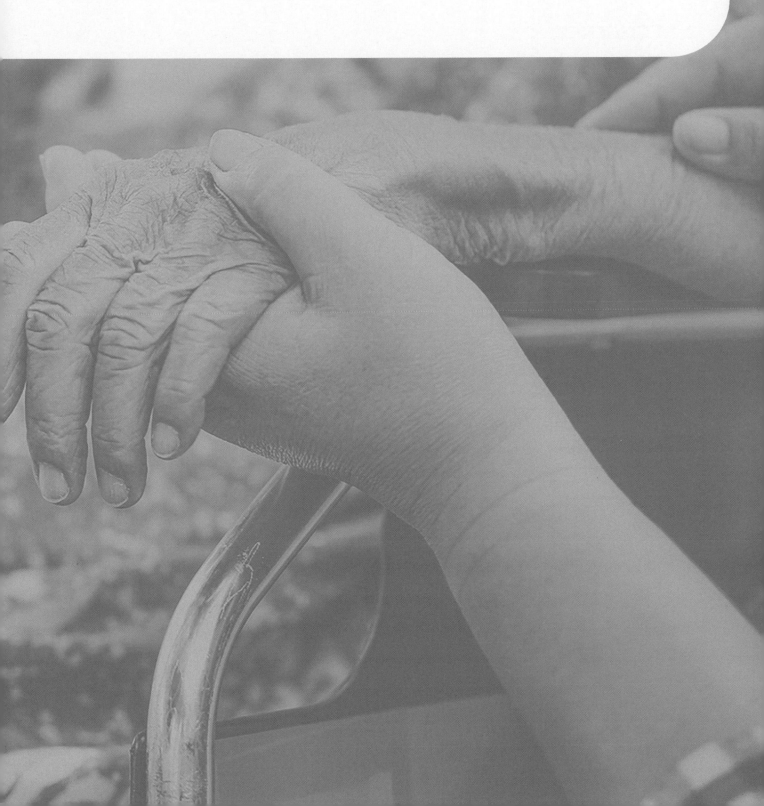

1. THE LAW AND THE AGED CARE SECTOR

(page 84 of Scott, Webb and Kostelnick, 5th edition)

In Australia, laws are enacted by governments (state or federal) as statutes or legislation. What legislation specifically relates to the work of carers in the aged care sector?

_____

_____

_____

_____

_____

2. NEGLIGENCE

(page 84 of Scott, Webb and Kostelnick, 5th edition)

To establish negligence, four conditions must all be proved:

1. _____

   _____

2. _____

   _____

3. _____

   _____

4. _____

   _____

Activity 1

You take Mrs Smith to the shower. Her care plan states that you must fasten a lap restraint around her, as she is at risk of falling out of the commode chair. You are very busy and forget to secure the lap restraint. While she is in the shower, Mrs Smith asks you to pass her the shampoo. As you are walking to the other end of the bathroom, Mrs Smith leans forward and falls out of the commode chair, fracturing her femur. She is admitted to hospital for surgery.

Looking at the four elements of negligence, are you negligent in your care of Mrs Smith? Why, or why not?

_____

_____

_____

_____

_____

Has your standard of care fallen below the standard required of a care worker? Yes or no? How do you determine the standard of care required by care workers?

_____

_____

_____

_____

Now reconsider the scenario above. Mrs Smith again falls out of the commode chair, but this time she is not injured. Are you negligent? Has your standard of care fallen below that required of a care worker?

_____

_____

_____

_____

3. DEFAMATION

(page 85 of Scott, Webb and Kostelnick, 5th edition)

What is the difference between slander and libel?

_____

_____

_____

4. ASSAULT AND BATTERY

(page 85 of Scott, Webb and Kostelnick, 5th edition)

What is the difference between assault and battery?

_____

_____

_____

What is the defence for assault and battery on a person?

_____

_____

_____

5. RESTRICTIVE PRACTICES

(pages 85–86 of Scott, Webb and Kostelnick, 5th edition)

What is meant by a 'restrictive practice'?

_____

_____

_____

In what circumstances can a restrictive practice be used?

_____

_____

_____

Name the different types of restraints that can be used, and give an example of each.

_____

_____

_____

_____

6. DOCUMENTATION AND RESTRICTIVE PRACTICES

What documentation is required before using a restrictive practice?

_____

_____

_____

7. MONITORING RESTRICTIVE PRACTICES

Documentation and records must be kept when using a restrictive practice. What documentation is required and who is responsible for completing this documentation?

_____

_____

_____

8. INFORMED CONSENT

(page 86 of Scott, Webb and Kostelnick, 5th edition)

What are the elements of informed consent?

_____

_____

_____

_____

_____

_____

_____

Who can give informed consent?

_____

_____

_____

_____

_____

_____

Valid Consent

For consent to be valid, the following criteria must exist:

• The person must have the legal capacity.

• Consent must be given freely.

• Consent must be specific – that is, it relates only to the treatment or procedure about which the client has been informed and has agreed to.

Activity 2

You are visiting one of your clients, Mr Jones, at his home. Mr Jones is of sound mind. He is complaining of chest pain and you are concerned that he might be having a heart attack. You ask Mr Jones if you can call an ambulance, but he refuses to go to hospital by ambulance.

Does Mr Jones have the right to withhold consent?

_____

_____

_____

_____

What should you do now?

_____

_____

_____

_____

9. DO NOT RESUSCITATE

(pages 86–87 of Scott, Webb and Kostelnick, 5th edition)

What elements do you need to consider when a client has a 'do not resuscitate' order in place?

_____

_____

_____

_____

10. DUTY OF CARE

(page 87 of Scott, Webb and Kostelnick, 5th edition)

What is meant by 'duty of care'?

_____

_____

_____

_____

Activity 3

You take Mrs Black to the shower. She is frail and confused. While you are attending to Mrs Black in the shower, Mr Bloomfield calls out that he is going to be sick. You rush off to get Mr Bloomfield a vomit bowl. When you get back, Mrs Black has fallen on the bathroom floor and hit her head.

Have you breached your duty of care? Give examples. How else could/should you have handled this situation?

_____

_____

_____

_____

11. VICARIOUS LIABILITY

(page 87 of Scott, Webb and Kostelnick, 5th edition)

What is meant by vicarious liability?

_____

_____

_____

_____

12. ABUSE

(pages 87 of Scott, Webb and Kostelnick, 5th edition)

What are the elements of abuse?

_____

_____

_____

_____

_____

13. ELDER ABUSE

(pages 87–88 of Scott, Webb and Kostelnick, 5th edition)

Read Box 3.1.

List the types of elder abuse experienced by older Australians and give an example of each type.

_____

_____

_____

_____

_____

_____

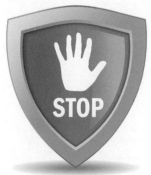

Figure 3.2 Stop elder abuse
iStockphoto/arcady_31

Activity 4

You are working in an aged care facility or community environment. You suspect one of your clients is being abused. The client tells you that the family members eat her Meals on Wheels meals, take her pension money and lock her in the home when they go out.

What does Australian legislation state about reporting elder abuse?

What steps must you take according to your employers policies and procedures?

_____

_____

_____

_____

_____

14. CONFIDENTIALITY

(page 88 of Scott, Webb and Kostelnick, 5th edition)

How can you maintain a client's confidentiality?

_____

_____

_____

_____

15. BULLYING AND HARASSMENT

(page 88 of Scott, Webb and Kostelnick, 5th edition)

What are some examples of bullying and harassment in the workplace?

_____

_____

_____

16. SEXUAL HARASSMENT

(page 89 of Scott, Webb and Kostelnick, 5th edition)

What are some examples of sexual harassment?

_____

_____

_____

_____

_____

_____

17. ETHICS AND THE AGED CARE SECTOR

(pages 89 of Scott, Webb and Kostelnick, 5th edition)

Read about ethics and ethical behaviour.

How can you as a care worker demonstrate ethical behaviours in the workplace?

_____

_____

_____

_____

_____

18. GUARDIANSHIP AND ENDURING POWER OF ATTORNEY

(page 90 of Scott, Webb and Kostelnick, 5th edition)

What decisions can a guardian make?

_____

_____

_____

_____

What is meant by 'enduring power of attorney'?

_____

_____

_____

_____

19. RESIDENTS' RIGHTS AND RESPONSIBILITIES

(page 90–93 of Scott, Webb and Kostelnick, 5th edition)

Read Box 3.2, Charter of Care Recipient Rights and Responsibilities.

Activity 5

Mrs Williams is 90 years old. She does not have any cognitive impairment. However, she has become increasingly frail and is at risk of falls. Mrs Williams walks with a walking frame. Her family members are worried that she might fall and don't want her walking anymore, but Mrs Williams wants to walk to the toilet and the dining room unaided.

What are Mrs Williams's rights?

_____

_____

_____

What strategies could you implement to make it safer for Mrs Williams to walk to the toilet and dining room?

_____

_____

_____

_____

20. RESIDENTS' RIGHTS TO MAKE PERSONAL CHOICES

(pages 92–93 of Scott, Webb and Kostelnick, 5th edition)

What personal choices can residents make?

_____

_____

_____

_____

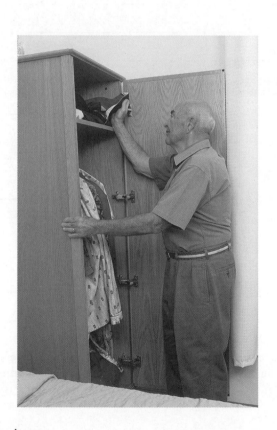

Figure 3.3 Providing a right to choose
(Sorrentino A & Gorek B 2003 Mosby's Textbook for Long-Term Care Assistants (4th edn), Mosby, St Louis.)

21. PRIVACY AND CONFIDENTIALITY

(page 92 of Scott, Webb and Kostelnick, 5th edition)

In addition to the privacy issues discussed earlier, residents have a right to personal privacy.

List all the things you can think of that relate to a resident's personal privacy.

_____

_____

_____

_____

_____

_____

22. DISPUTES AND GRIEVANCES

(page 92 of Scott, Webb and Kostelnick, 5th edition)

How do clients go about reporting disputes and grievances?

_____

_____

_____

_____

23. ADVANCE HEALTH DIRECTIVES

(page 86 of Scott, Webb and Kostelnick, 5th edition)

List at least three (3) things that a person may include in their Advance Health Directives.

_____

_____

_____

_____

Unit CHCDIV001:
Work with diverse people

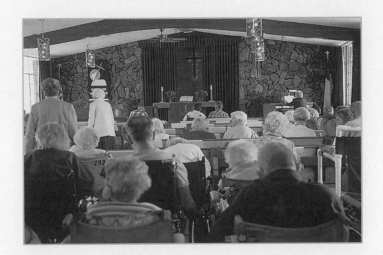

Figure 4.1 Cultural awareness
(Reproduced with permission from Sorrentino A & Gorek B (2011) Mosby's textbook for long-term care nursing assistants (6th edn) Mosby, St Louis)

Table of Contents

INTRODUCTION

This workbook relates to the unit **CHCDIV001: Work with diverse people**.

The workbook activities and final assessment tasks will enable you to:

- reflect on your own perspective
- appreciate diversity and inclusiveness, and their benefits
- communicate with people from diverse backgrounds and situations
- promote understanding across diverse groups.

To prepare for this unit and the assessment activities, we recommend that you first read Chapter 6 of Scott, Webb and Kostelnick, 5th edition, **Working with Australian Aboriginal and Torres Strait Islander Elders** and Chapter 8, **Working with older people from diverse cultural backgrounds**.

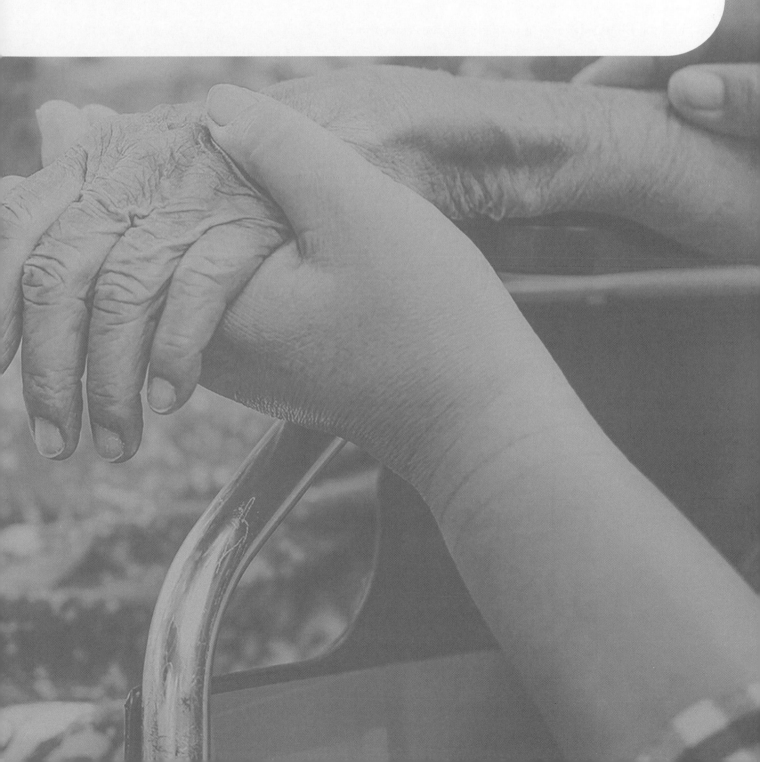

1. HISTORY OF MULTICULTURALISM IN AUSTRALIA

(pages 154–155 of Scott, Webb and Kostelnick, 5th edition)

The original people in Australia are the Aboriginal and Torres Strait Islander peoples.

After the introduction of the *Migration Act 1958*, who were the main immigrants to Australia?

_____

_____

_____

_____

_____

Since the 1990s, where do most of our migrants come from?

_____

_____

_____

2. CULTURE, RACE AND ETHNICITY

(pages 155–156 of Scott, Webb and Kostelnick, 5th edition)

What is meant by 'culture'?

_____

_____

_____

_____

_____

What is meant by 'race'?

_____

_____

_____

What is meant by 'ethnicity'?

_____

_____

_____

_____

3. CULTURAL AWARENESS AND CULTURAL SENSITIVITY

(page 156 of Scott, Webb and Kostelnick, 5th edition)

Activity 1

If you are caring for a client in an aged care facility or community setting, that client has the right to culturally appropriate care.

What could you do to ensure that your client receives culturally appropriate care?

_____

_____

_____

_____

_____

_____

4. CULTURAL SAFETY AND THE CARER

(page 156 of Scott, Webb and Kostelnick, 5th edition)

Consideration must also be given to the cultural safety of the carer. If you are asked to care for a client or to undertake any activities that you believe will compromise your cultural safety, you have the right to refuse to undertake them.

Can you think of an example where you might refuse to undertake an activity?

_____

_____

_____

_____

_____

5. ATTITUDES TO AGEING

(page 156 of Scott, Webb and Kostelnick, 5th edition)

Attitudes to ageing vary across cultures. Many migrant groups also have views and practices that may differ from your own.

Activity 2

Break into small groups. List three attitudes various cultures have when it comes to caring for the elderly. Once you have made your list, the trainer will ask you to present to the class for discussion.

_____

_____

_____

6. ADDRESSING THE OLDER PERSON

(page 156 of Scott, Webb and Kostelnick, 5th edition)

Always check with your client how they wish to be addressed.

Think of some clients you have cared for and write down some examples of how they told you they wished to be addressed.

_____

_____

_____

_____

7. TOUCHING

(page 157 of Scott, Webb and Kostelnick, 5th edition)

Can you think of some examples of when it is *not* culturally appropriate to touch a client, and some examples of when it *is* culturally appropriate to touch a client?

_____

_____

_____

_____

_____

8. FAMILY ATTITUDES

(page 157 of Scott, Webb and Kostelnick, 5th edition)

Many cultural groups hold strong beliefs about caring for the older person.

Can you list some beliefs that family members from another cultural group might hold about caring for the older person?

_____

_____

_____

_____

_____

9. LANGUAGE

(pages 157–158 of Scott, Webb and Kostelnick, 5th edition)

Read the section relating to languages spoken in Australia. As people age, they can lose some of their language skills or revert back to their native language.

Activity 3

Break into small groups. Write down various ways you could communicate with someone who speaks a language other than English.

_____

_____

_____

_____

_____

Also give some examples of strategies the group members have used in the workplace to communicate effectively with people speaking a language other than English.

_____

_____

_____

_____

_____

10. DRESS

(page 158 of Scott, Webb and Kostelnick, 5th edition)

Many cultures have specific dress codes that must be followed.

List some dress codes that you have come across as an aged care worker.

_____

_____

_____

11. DIET

(page 158 of Scott, Webb and Kostelnick, 5th edition)

Your client may be used to a diet that is different from what is generally considered normal within mainstream Australia.

Activity 4

Families will sometimes bring in food for the client in a community setting, or you might need to cook the client's meal. What are some rules and regulations for cooking food, or for family bringing in food from home, that you must adhere to?

_____

_____

_____

_____

_____

Think of some different ethnic/religious groups and write down what foods they are and are not permitted to eat.

_____

_____

_____

_____

_____

12. RELIGION

(pages 158–161 of Scott, Webb and Kostelnick, 5th edition)

It is important to respect clients' spiritual beliefs, needs and practices.

Activity 5

Break into small groups. Think of four different types of religions practised in Australia. In the second column, write what you could do to assist your client to practise their religious beliefs, whether they be in a residential aged care facility or in the community.

Religion	How you can assist the client to practise their religion
1	
2	
3	
4	

13. SERVICES AVAILABLE FOR PEOPLE FROM CULTURALLY AND LINGUISTICALLY DIVERSE BACKGROUNDS (CALD)

(page 162 of Scott, Webb and Kostelnick, 5th edition)

When you care for a client from a culturally and linguistically diverse background, a number of organisations and services can assist you to provide appropriate care.

_____
_____
_____
_____
_____

14. ABORIGINAL AND TORRES STRAIT ISLANDER CULTURE

(page 130 of Scott, Webb and Kostelnick, 5th edition)

Across Australia, there are hundreds of different Aboriginal nations.

Read Chapter 6 of Scott, Webb and Kostelnick, 5th edition, especially Table 6.1 on pages 133–135.

Activity 6

At the time of colonisation the Indigenous Australians were a fit, healthy people. Since colonisation, they have suffered a lot of health problems. Can you list four of the health problems faced by the Aboriginal and Torres Strait Islander peoples?

_____
_____
_____
_____

When caring for Aboriginal and Torres Strait Islander peoples, we often refer to 'women's' and 'men's' business. What is meant by this term? How can you ensure culturally appropriate care for these clients?

_____
_____
_____
_____
_____

Unit CHCCOM005:
Communicate and work in health or community services

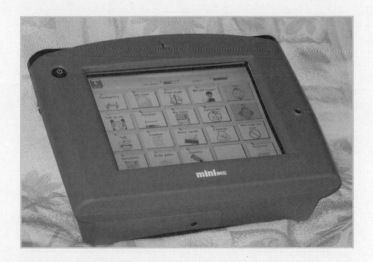

Figure 5.1 Picture board used to communicate
(© Link Assistive, www.linkassistive.com.)

Table of Contents

INTRODUCTION

This workbook relates to the unit **CHCCOM005: Communicate and work in health or community services**.

The workbook activities and final assessment tasks will enable you to:

- communicate effectively with people
- collaborate with colleagues
- address constraints to communication
- report problems to supervisor
- complete workplace correspondence and documentation
- contribute to continuous improvement.

To prepare for this unit and the assessment activities, we recommend that you first read Chapter 9 of Scott, Webb and Kostelnick, 5th edition, **Interpersonal communication and care**.

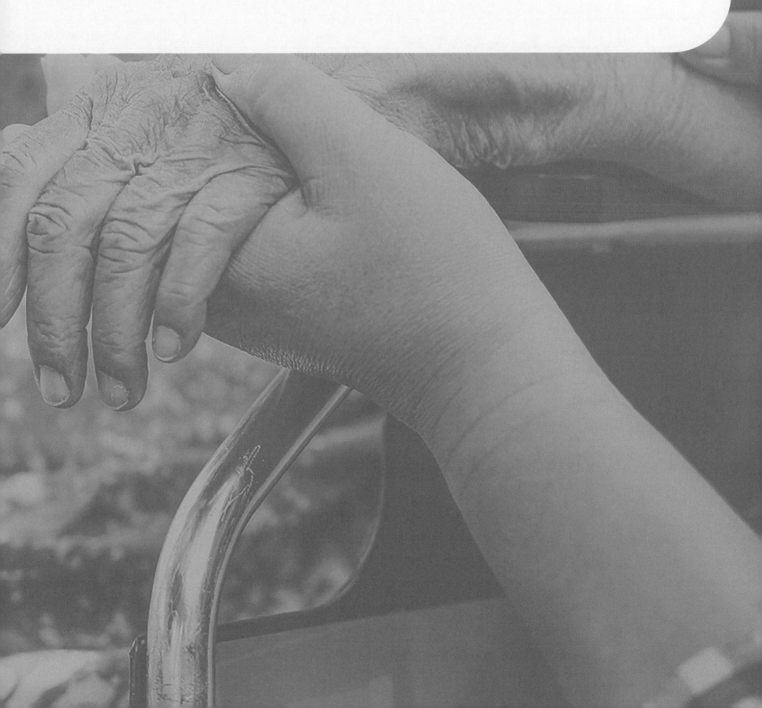

1. COMMUNICATING EFFECTIVELY WITH CLIENTS

(page 166 of Scott, Webb and Kostelnick, 5th edition)

You communicate with clients every time you give care.

Effective communication takes place when you:

_____

_____

_____

_____

_____

_____

_____

_____

_____

_____

_____

_____

_____

Communicating with Other Staff in the Workplace

Give five (5) examples of how you can communicate with someone who only has written communication skills.

_____

_____

_____

_____

_____

_____

_____

_____

_____

_____

_____

_____

_____

2. VERBAL COMMUNICATION

(page 168 of Scott, Webb and Kostelnick, 5th edition)

What are the rules to follow when speaking with a client?

_____

_____

_____

_____

_____

_____

_____

_____

_____

_____

3. WRITTEN COMMUNICATION

(page 169 of Scott, Webb and Kostelnick, 5th edition)

How do you communicate with a person who only has written communication skills?

_____

_____

_____

_____

_____

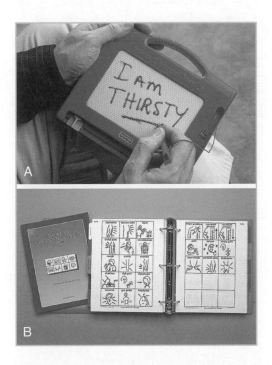

Figure 5.2 Communication aids. **A.** Magic slate. **B.** Communication board
(A: Reproduced with permission from Sorrentino A & Gorek B (2011). Mosby's textbook for long-term care nursing assistants (6th edn). Mosby, St Louis. B: Sorrentino A & Gorek B, Mosby's Textbook for Long-Term Care Assistants (4th edn), Mosby, St Louis.)

4. NON-VERBAL COMMUNICATION

(pages 166–168 of Scott, Webb and Kostelnick, 5th edition)

Some types of non-verbal communication are:

_____

_____

_____

_____

_____

Why should you always be aware of your own non-verbal communication when addressing a client?

_____

_____

_____

_____

_____

Touch

Touch is an important part of non-verbal communication. When is it appropriate to touch someone, and when is it not appropriate? How do you know if someone likes to be touched or not?

_____

_____

_____

Body language

Your actions send messages that are often more powerful than words. Your residents also send messages via their body language. A resident who might not be able to verbalise pain may hold their side to indicate hip pain.

Describe some other types of messages people send via their body language.

_____

_____

_____

_____

_____

5. COMMUNICATION METHODS

(pages 168–169 of Scott, Webb and Kostelnick, 5th edition)

Listening

What are effective listening skills?

_____

_____

_____

_____

_____

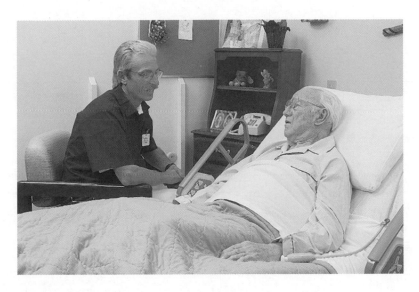

Figure 5.3 Listening skills
(Sorrentino A & Gorek B, Mosby's Textbook for Long-Term Care Assistants (4th edn), Mosby, St Louis.)

Paraphrasing

Paraphrasing is restating the person's message in your own words.

Activity 1

Break up into groups of two and take it in turns to tell each other something. The person listening will paraphrase the message back to the other person in their own words. This exercise might seem easy, but let's see how well we can paraphrase. Suggest why the message was misinterpreted, if that was the case.

_____

_____

_____

_____

_____

Direct Questions

Direct questions focus on certain information you need to know. Some have 'yes' or 'no' answers, while others require the person to give more information.

What types of clients would respond best to direct questions?

_____

_____

_____

_____

_____

Open-Ended Questions

Open-ended questions lead or invite the person to share their thoughts, feelings or ideas.

Some examples of open-ended questions are:

_____

_____

_____

_____

Clarifying

Clarifying ensures you understand the message. How can you clarify with a person that they have understood the message you are trying to convey to them?

_____

_____

_____

_____

_____

Focusing

Some clients with a cognitive impairment cannot focus on one topic.

Activity 2

Think of someone with a cognitive impairment who has trouble focusing on a topic. How can you get the person to focus?

_____

_____

_____

_____

6. COMMUNICATION BARRIERS

(page 169 of Scott, Webb and Kostelnick, 5th edition)

Communication barriers prevent us from sending and receiving messages. Some barriers to communication are:

_____

_____

_____

_____

_____

7. CARING FOR THE PERSON

(pages 169–171 of Scott, Webb and Kostelnick, 5th edition)

How you care for the person holistically (treating something or someone as a 'whole' – physically, socially, psychologically, emotionally and spiritually) is an important aspect of communication.

Activity 3

What do you think is meant by treating the person as a 'whole'? Give five examples of how you treat a person as a 'whole'.

_____

_____

_____

_____

_____

_____

_____

_____

8. NEEDS

(page 170 of Scott, Webb and Kostelnick, 5th edition)

Take some time to look at Fig. 5.4, Maslow's hierarchy of needs.

For each need, list some examples.

Physiological needs:

_____

_____

_____

_____

Need for safety:

_____

_____

_____

_____

_____

Need for love and belonging:

_____

_____

_____

_____

_____

Need for esteem:

_____

_____

_____

_____

_____

Need for self-actualisation:

_____

_____

_____

_____

_____

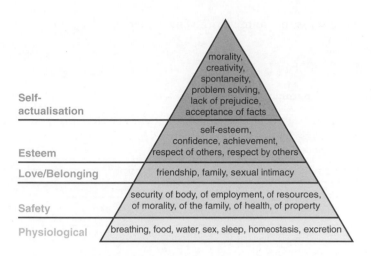

Figure 5.4 Maslow's Hierarchy of Needs
(Created by J. Finkelstein CC-BY-SA-3.0.)

9. CULTURE AND RELIGION

(pages 171–172 of Scott, Webb and Kostelnick, 5th edition)

Religion influences a person's health and illness practice. It may affect their belief about diet, healing, days of worship, birth and death.

What can a residential aged care facility/community facility do to ensure that clients are able to observe their religious and cultural practices?

_____

_____

_____

_____

10. EFFECTS OF ILLNESS AND DISABILITY ON COMMUNICATION

(pages 172–174 of Scott, Webb and Kostelnick, 5th edition)

A person might acquire a disability from birth through to old age. If someone with a disability is not able to verbally communicate how they feel, they might do so by exhibiting behaviours and emotions.

Name some examples where you have seen a person with a disability behave when they have not been able to express how they feel. How can you assist a person with a disability to express how they feel? For example, Jim comes home from working at the Botanical Gardens and is very angry and abusive towards his flatmates. A physiotherapist assesses Jim and finds he has back pain made worse by the heavy work in the garden. She treats his back pain and gives him some exercises to do, and Jim's behaviour improves.

_____

_____

_____

_____

_____

_____

Read Box 9.1 on page 173, and discuss the content with your trainer and the group.

11. RESIDENTS AND CLIENTS

(pages 173–175 of Scott, Webb and Kostelnick, 5th edition)

Residents of care facilities have often been treated as sick, dependent people. This reduces quality of life and aids dependency. How can you enable a resident to be more independent?

_____

_____

_____

Confused and Disoriented Residents

What are some common causes of confusion in an older client?

_____

_____

_____

_____

_____

High-Care Clients

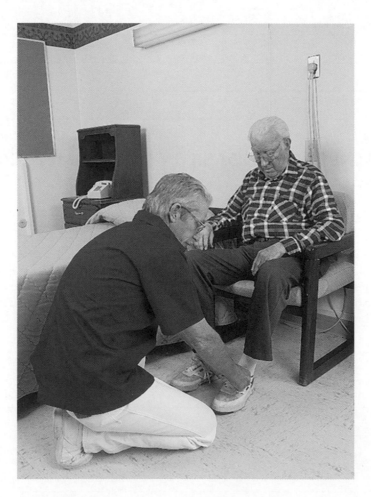

Figure 5.5 Services for older adults
(Sorrentino A & Gorek B, Mosby's Textbook for Long-Term Care Assistants (4th edn), Mosby, St Louis.)

Activity 4

Some clients require assistance with all their activities of daily living. They may be confused and disoriented as well. They might understand what you are saying but cannot communicate their needs. How would you, as a care worker, ensure that your client's needs are being met?

_____

_____

_____

_____

_____

_____

_____

_____

How might the needs of a client with mental illness differ from other clients?

_____

_____

_____

_____

_____

_____

_____

_____

We will talk about palliative care later in the workbook. Briefly describe how the needs of a terminally ill client might differ from those of clients you normally care for.

_____

_____

_____

_____

_____

12. COMMUNICATION AND CHANGED BEHAVIOURS

(pages 174–175 of Scott, Webb and Kostelnick, 5th edition)

Some behaviours exhibited by clients might be new, and some might be the client's personality. Behaviours often convey something the person wishes to communicate.

Activity 5

For each of the challenging behaviours listed below, write why you think the person might be exhibiting this behaviour and what strategies can be put into place to manage the behaviour. Read Box 9.2 on page 175.

Anger:

_____

_____

_____

_____

Demanding behaviour:

_____

_____

_____

Self-centred behaviour:

_____

_____

_____

_____

Aggressive behaviour:

_____

_____

_____

_____

Withdrawal:

_____

_____

_____

_____

Inappropriate sexual behaviour:

_____

_____

_____

_____

The Client who is Comatose

(page 175 of Scott, Webb and Kostelnick, 5th edition)

The unconscious person can often hear, and feel sensations such as touch and pain. They might grimace when in pain.

How would you communicate and care for a person who is unconscious?

_____

_____

_____

_____

_____

_____

_____

13. FAMILY AND FRIENDS

(pages 175–176 of Scott, Webb and Kostelnick, 5th edition)

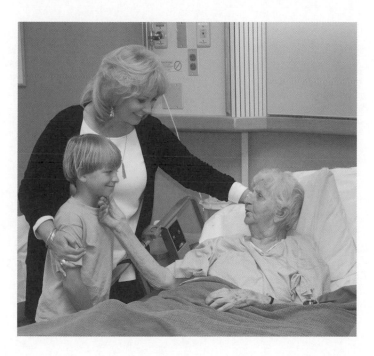

Figure 5.6 Family visits
(© 2010 Jupiterimages Corporation.)

Why is it important to communicate with a client's family and friends?

_____

_____

_____

_____

_____

_____

14. DOCUMENTATION AND CONTINUOUS IMPROVEMENT

_____

_____

_____

_____

_____

_____

_____

6a

Unit CHCCCS041:
Recognise healthy body systems

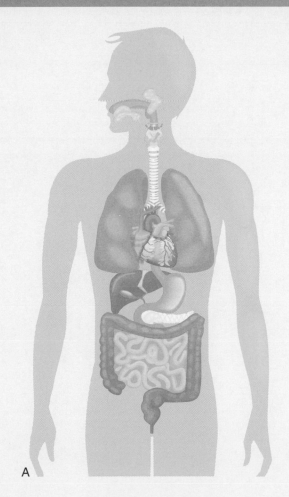

A

Figure 6a.1 The human body
(iStockphoto/Netta07)

Table of Contents

INTRODUCTION

This workbook relates to the unit **CHCCCS041: Recognise healthy body systems**.

The workbook activities and final assessment tasks will enable you to:

- work with information about the human body
- recognise and promote ways to support healthy functioning of the body.

To prepare for this unit and the assessment activities, we recommend that you first read Chapter 10 of Scott, Webb and Kostelnick, 5th edition, **The human body in health and disease**.

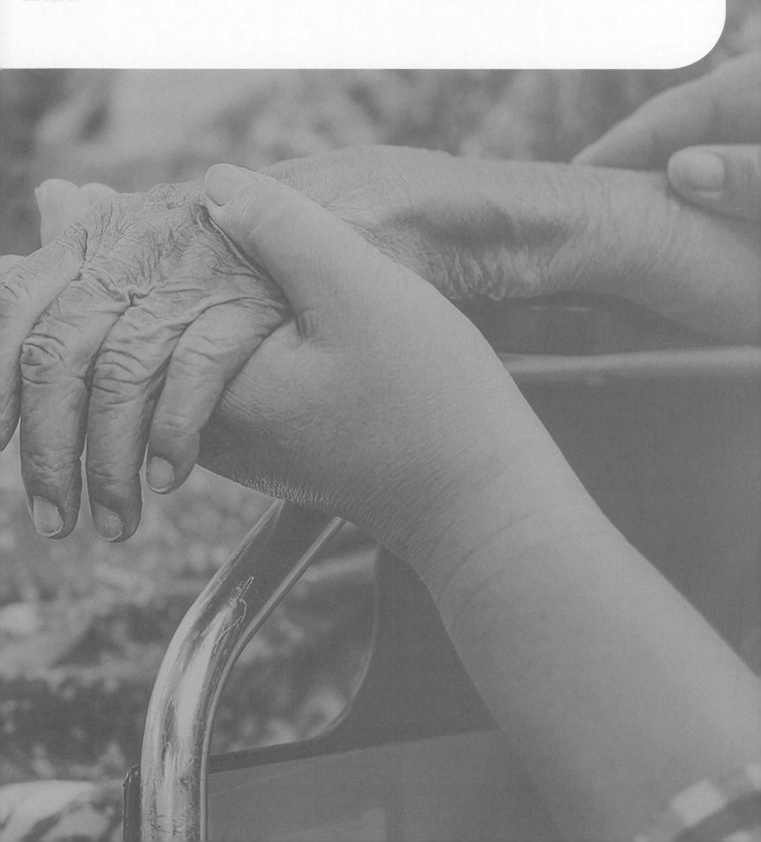

1. CELLS, TISSUES AND ORGANS

(pages 180–181 of Scott, Webb and Kostelnick, 5th edition)

The human body can be classified into six different levels of organisation (refer to Fig. 10.1 in Scott, Webb and Kostelnick, 5th edition). Give a brief explanation on the functions of each part of the cell.

1. Chemical

_____

_____

_____

2. Cellular

_____

_____

_____

Refer to Fig. 10.3 in Scott, Webb and Kostelnick, 5th edition.

3. Tissues

_____

_____

4. Organs

_____

_____

5. Organ system

_____

_____

6. Whole body system

_____

_____

Systems are formed by groups of organs working together to perform special functions. For example, the heart is part of the cardiovascular system. Below is a list of organ systems. Complete the table below by naming an organ and its function for each organ system.

Organ	Organ system	Function
	Integumentary	
	Musculoskeletal	
	Nervous	
	Cardiovascular	
	Respiratory	
	Digestive	
	Urinary	
	Reproductive	
	Endocrine	
	Immune	

2. INTEGUMENTARY SYSTEM

(pages 181–185 and Fig. 10.4 of Scott, Webb and Kostelnick, 5th edition)

Skin functions

The functions of the skin are:

_____

_____

_____

_____

_____

_____

_____

Skin Changes due to Ageing

Name four changes that occur in the integumentary system due to ageing, and identify strategies for maintaining a healthy integumentary system.

1 _____

_____

2 _____

_____

3 _____

_____

4 _____

_____

Skin Disorders

(pages 184–185 of Scott, Webb and Kostelnick, 5th edition)

Name a common skin condition that may occur in your care recipient, and suggest some prevention strategies.

_____

_____

_____

_____

3. MUSCULOSKELETAL SYSTEM

Musculoskeletal Functions

(pages 185–187 and Figs 10.8, 10.10 and 10.11 of Scott, Webb and Kostelnick, 5th edition)

The functions of the musculoskeletal system are:

_____

_____

_____

_____

_____

_____

_____

_____

_____

Musculoskeletal Changes due to Ageing

(pages 187 of Scott, Webb and Kostelnick, 5th edition)

List four changes that occur in the musculoskeletal system due to ageing, and identify one strategy for each of the four changes to assist in maintaining a healthy musculoskeletal system.

_____

_____

_____

_____

_____

_____

_____

_____

_____

Activity 1

Mrs Andrews is 86 years old, and suffering from osteoarthritis in her knees and hips. She had a right hip replacement three years ago. She loves to go for walks, to work in the garden and to meet friends for coffee. However, these tasks are becoming increasingly difficult and painful, and Mrs Andrews is feeling very socially isolated. She is also worried that if she goes out she might fall. As a carer in the community or in residential care, what strategies could you put into place to manage her pain, mobility and social isolation?

Pain management:

_____

_____

_____

_____

Mobility/falls management:

_____

_____

_____

_____

Suggestions for reducing social isolation:

_____

_____

_____

_____

Musculoskeletal Conditions

(pages 187–190 of Scott, Webb and Kostelnick, 5th edition)

Select one condition – osteoarthritis, rheumatoid arthritis or osteoporosis – and answer the questions below.

A brief outline of the condition

_____

_____

_____

_____

_____

What are the signs and symptoms of this condition?

_____

_____

_____

_____

_____

What strategies can you put into place to assist people with this condition with their activities of daily living?

_____

_____

_____

_____

_____

4. NERVOUS SYSTEM

(pages 195–198 and Figs 10.27 and 10.28 of Scott, Webb and Kostelnick, 5th edition)

Nervous System Functions

The functions of the nervous system are:

_____

_____

_____

_____

_____

Nervous System Changes due to Ageing

(page 198 of Scott, Webb and Kostelnick, 5th edition)

List three changes that occur in the nervous system due to ageing, and identify one condition that may occur for each of the three changes.

_____

_____

_____

_____

_____

_____

_____

Nervous System Disorders

(pages 198–201 of Scott, Webb and Kostelnick, 5th edition)

Cerebrovascular accident (stroke) is a common cause of disability among older people.

List the main causes or risk factors for a stroke:

_____

_____

_____

_____

_____

_____

List at least three effects that a stroke can have on a person:

_____

_____

_____

What are the signs and symptoms of Parkinson's disease?

_____

_____

_____

_____

_____

Provide a brief description of multiple sclerosis.

_____

_____

_____

_____

_____

Nervous System – Special Senses

(pages 201–208 and Figs 10.34 and 10.35 of Scott, Webb and Kostelnick, 5th edition)

The five main senses are sight, hearing, taste, smell and touch.

Activity 2

Mr Carson is 92 years old and has multiple sensory deficits including cataracts, hearing impairment and loss of taste and smell. List at least 10 strategies you would need to implement when assisting Mr Carson with his activities of daily living and socialising.

Strategies to implement to assist Mr Carson:

_____

_____

_____

_____

_____

_____

_____

_____

_____

_____

_____

_____

Nervous System – Special Senses Disorders (Eyes)

Glaucoma (brief description):

_____

_____

_____

_____

_____

_____

_____

Cataracts (brief description):

_____

_____

_____

_____

_____

_____

_____

Nervous System – Special Senses Disorders (Ears)

Hearing loss is common in older people but not all older people have a hearing impairment.

The main causes of chronic hearing loss are:

_____

_____

_____

_____

_____

_____

The main causes of temporary hearing loss are:

_____

_____

_____

_____

_____

List at least 10 tips for communicating with a person with a hearing impairment:

_____

_____

_____

_____

_____

_____

_____

_____

_____

_____

_____

_____

A hearing aid picks up sound and amplifies it for the wearer. It does not correct a hearing problem (refer to Fig. 10.36 on page 204, Scott, Webb and Kostelnick, 5th edition).

List all the steps required when caring for hearing aids:

_____

_____

_____

_____

_____

_____

_____

_____

_____

_____

5. CIRCULATORY SYSTEM

(pages 208–211 and Fig. 10.47 of Scott, Webb and Kostelnick, 5th edition)

What are the main organs of the circulatory system?

_____

_____

_____

_____

_____

_____

_____

_____

Cardiovascular Functions

What are the main functions of the cardiovascular system?

_____

_____

_____

_____

_____

_____

_____

Cardiovascular Changes due to Ageing

(pages 211–212 of Scott, Webb and Kostelnick, 5th edition)

As a person ages, changes take place in their cardiovascular system. Underneath each heading, write one change that occurs and how this change will impact on an older person.

Heart changes:

_____

_____

_____

Blood vessel changes:

_____

_____

_____

Blood changes:

_____

_____

_____

Cardiovascular Disorders

(pages 212–214 of Scott, Webb and Kostelnick, 5th edition)

Hypertension

If a person has hypertension, what factors cannot be changed?

_____

_____

_____

If a person has hypertension, what lifestyle/preventative factors can be changed?

_____

_____

_____

Coronary Artery Disease

What lifestyle changes can a person make to prevent coronary artery disease and heart attack?

_____

_____

_____

_____

_____

_____

6. RESPIRATORY SYSTEM

(pages 214–215 and Fig. 10.53 of Scott, Webb and Kostelnick, 5th edition)

Respiratory Functions

Fill in the gaps using data from the table underneath.

The respiratory system brings _____ into the lungs and eliminates _____. The process is called _____. This involves _____ (breathing in) and _____ (breathing out). Air enters the body though the _____ and then passes into the _____ (throat). Air passes from the larynx into the _____. From there, it travels to the right and left _____. These divide into _____ eventually ending in one-celled air sacs called _____. It is here that _____ and _____ are exchanged between the alveoli and capillaries.

alveoli	bronchi
bronchioles	carbon dioxide
carbon dioxide	expiration
inspiration	nose
oxygen	oxygen
pharynx	respiration
trachea	

Respiratory Changes due to Ageing

(pages 215–216 of Scott, Webb and Kostelnick, 5th edition)

List three aged-related changes that occur in the respiratory system.

_____

_____

_____

_____

Respiratory Disorders

(pages 216–218 of Scott, Webb and Kostelnick, 5th edition)

Chronic Obstructive Airway Disease (COAD)

Definition:

_____

_____

_____

_____

What are the main causes of COAD?

_____

_____

_____

_____

7. DIGESTIVE SYSTEM

(pages 217–218 and Fig. 10.56 of Scott, Webb and Kostelnick, 5th edition)

Digestive Functions

List at least three functions of the digestive system.

_____

_____

_____

Digestive Changes due to Ageing

(page 219 of Scott, Webb and Kostelnick, 5th edition)

Name four aged-related changes that occur in the digestive system, and identify one strategy for each change to assist in maintaining a healthy digestive system.

_____

_____

_____

_____

_____

_____

_____

Digestive Disorders

(pages 219–220 of Scott, Webb and Kostelnick, 5th edition)

Give a brief description of each of the following three digestive disorders in people and one strategy for each disorder to manage it.

Vomiting:

_____

_____

_____

_____

Gastric Oesophageal Reflux Disease (GORD):

_____

_____

_____

_____

Peptic ulcer:

_____

_____

_____

_____

8. URINARY SYSTEM

(page 221 and Fig. 10.59 of Scott, Webb and Kostelnick, 5th edition)

Urinary functions

List the two main functions of the urinary system.

_____

_____

_____

_____

Give a brief description of the function of the parts of the urinary system listed below:

Nephron:

_____

_____

Ureter:

_____

_____

Bladder:

_____

_____

Urine:

_____

_____

Urinary Changes due to Ageing

(page 221 of Scott, Webb and Kostelnick, 5th edition)

Describe three changes that occur in the urinary system due to ageing.

_____

_____

_____

_____

_____

Urinary Disorders

(page 222 of Scott, Webb and Kostelnick, 5th edition)

Urinary Tract Infections (UTIs)

UTIs are common in older people.

List three causes of UTIs in older people:

_____

_____

_____

_____

Renal Failure

In renal failure, waste products are not removed from the blood and the body retains fluid. Renal failure may be acute or chronic.

Give a brief description of the following conditions.

Acute renal failure:

_____

_____

_____

_____

Chronic renal failure:

_____

_____

_____

_____

9. REPRODUCTIVE SYSTEM

(pages 222–224 and Figs 10.61 and 10.62 of Scott, Webb and Kostelnick, 5th edition)

Reproductive Functions

What is the main function of the reproductive system?

_____

_____

_____

_____

Reproductive Changes due to Ageing

(page 225 of Scott, Webb and Kostelnick, 5th edition)

Describe the changes that occur in the reproductive system due to ageing.

Male	Female

Reproductive Disorders

(pages 225–226 of Scott, Webb and Kostelnick, 5th edition)

Give a brief description of the two main female reproductive disorders.

Ovarian cancer:

_____

_____

_____

Breast cancer:

_____

_____

_____

_____

Briefly describe the two main male reproductive disorders common in men as they become older.

Benign prostatic hyperplasia (BPH):

_____

_____

_____

Prostate cancer:

_____

_____

_____

10. ENDOCRINE SYSTEM

(pages 226–227 and Fig. 10.65 of Scott, Webb and Kostelnick, 5th edition)

Endocrine Functions

The endocrine system is made up of glands that secrete hormones. Give a brief description of one hormone relating to the endocrine system and the function of this hormone.

_____

_____

_____

_____

_____

Give a brief description of the term metabolism.

_____

_____

_____

_____

_____

Endocrine Changes due to Ageing

(page 227 of Scott, Webb and Kostelnick, 5th edition)

Describe the main aged-related change that occurs to the endocrine system.

_____

_____

_____

Endocrine Disorders

(page 227 of Scott, Webb and Kostelnick, 5th edition)

One of the most common endocrine disorders is type 2 diabetes.

Briefly describe what type 2 diabetes is and how it affects people.

_____

_____

_____

_____

_____

Describe risk factors for diabetes, and identify strategies for managing these risk factors.

_____

_____

_____

_____

_____

_____

_____

_____

What lifestyle changes must a person living with type 2 diabetes make?

_____

_____

_____

_____

11. IMMUNE SYSTEM

(pages 227–228 of Scott, Webb and Kostelnick, 5th edition)

Immune Functions

The immune system protects the body from diseases and infections and provides it with immunity. List some of the special cells and substances that function to produce immunity.

_____

_____

_____

_____

Immune Changes due to Ageing

(page 228 of Scott, Webb and Kostelnick, 5th edition)

As the body ages, it becomes less efficient at protecting itself from disease. List some of the reasons that an older person is more at risk of infection.

_____

_____

_____

_____

As a support worker, list at least four strategies you can employ to reduce the spread of infection.

_____

_____

_____

_____

Immune Disorders

(page 229 of Scott, Webb and Kostelnick, 5th edition)

The older person has a reduced resistance to infectious and autoimmune diseases. List some of the conditions they are at risk of contracting.

_____

_____

_____

_____

Unit CHCCCS041:
Recognise healthy body systems: health assessment

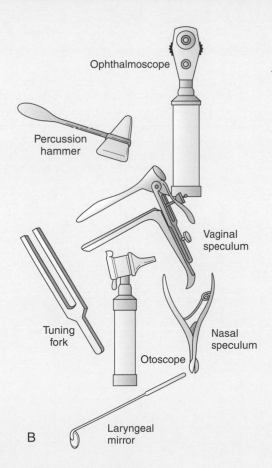

Ophthalmoscope

Percussion
hammer

Vaginal
speculum

Tuning
fork

Nasal
speculum

Otoscope

B   Laryngeal
mirror

Figure 6b.1 Instruments used for physical examination.
(Sorrentino A & Gorek B 2010 Mosby's Textbook for Long-Term Care Assistants (6th edn), Mosby, St Louis.)

Table of Contents

INTRODUCTION

This workbook relates to the unit **CHCCCS041: Recognise healthy body systems**.

The workbook activities and final assessment tasks will enable you to:

- work with information about the human body
- recognise and promote ways to support healthy functioning of the body.

To prepare for this unit and the assessment activities, we recommend that you first read Chapter 11 of Scott, Webb and Kostelnick, 5th edition, **Health assessment**.

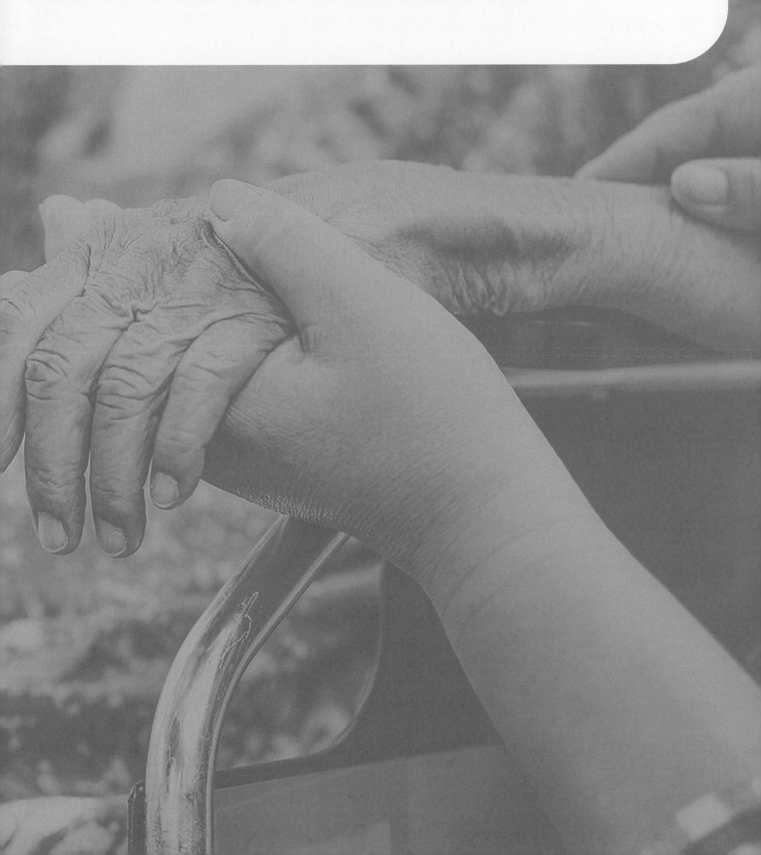

1. PHYSICAL EXAMINATION

(page 234 of Scott, Webb and Kostelnick, 5th edition)

Why might a care recipient need to undergo a physical examination?

_____

_____

_____

_____

_____

_____

_____

_____

_____

_____

Activity 1

Next to the name of a piece of equipment listed below, state what it is used for.

Ophthalmoscope:

_____

_____

_____

Otoscope:

_____

_____

_____

Percussion hammer:

_____

_____

_____

Vaginal speculum:

_____

_____

_____

Nasal speculum:

_____

_____

_____

Tuning fork:

_____

_____

_____

Laryngeal mirror:

_____

_____

_____

Tympanic membrane thermometer:

_____

_____

_____

Stethoscope:

_____

_____

_____

Sphygmomanometer:

_____

_____

_____

What support might be required from a support worker during a physical examination?

_____

_____

_____

_____

2. VITAL SIGNS

(pages 236–246 of Scott, Webb and Kostelnick, 5th edition)

List the types of vital signs you might measure. Next to each vital sign write in the normal values you would expect to see in an adult. What can this show about the person?

_____

_____

_____

_____

_____

_____

_____

3. WHERE DO YOU REPORT VITAL SIGNS?

(pages 236–251 of Scott, Webb and Kostelnick, 5th edition)

_____

_____

_____

_____

What steps do you take if a person's vital signs are not within the normal range?

_____

_____

_____

Activity 2

In residential aged care, you might not always need to take vital signs on a regular basis. However, in what situations do you think you might need to take someone's vital signs?

_____

_____

_____

_____

_____

4. BODY TEMPERATURE

(pages 237 of Scott, Webb and Kostelnick, 5th edition)

What is body temperature?

_____

_____

_____

_____

_____

_____

_____

Activity 3

List the types of thermometers that measure body temperature.

_____

_____

_____

_____

_____

_____

_____

_____

When should you not use an oral thermometer to take a person's temperature?

_____

_____

_____

Practical Exercise: Taking Body Temperature

Refer to the box 'Delegation guidelines: Taking temperatures' on page 237.

What is your role as a support worker when it comes to taking temperatures? What steps should you take?

_____

_____

5. PULSE

(pages 238–242 and Fig. 11.7 of Scott, Webb and Kostelnick, 5th edition)

Where on the body can you take someone's pulse?

_____

_____

_____

_____

Activity 4

1 What is the normal pulse rate of an adult?

_____

_____

_____

_____

2 What is meant by the terms 'tachycardia' and 'bradycardia'?

_____

_____

_____

_____

3 Why is the rhythm and force of the pulse important?

_____

_____

_____

_____

_____

6. STETHOSCOPE

(pages 243–245 and Fig. 11.8 of Scott, Webb and Kostelnick, 5th edition)

What are stethoscopes used for?

_____
_____
_____
_____
_____

Activity 5

Practical Exercise: Taking a Radial Pulse

Look at the Delegation guidelines 'Taking a pulse' on page 242. What do the guidelines outline you should do?

_____
_____
_____

7. RESPIRATION

(page 242 of Scott, Webb and Kostelnick, 5th edition)

Under what circumstances would you need to check a person's respirations?

_____
_____
_____
_____

Activity 6

Look at the box 'Delegating guidelines: Counting respirations' on page 242. What do the guidelines state a support worker should do when counting respirations?

_____
_____
_____
_____

8. BLOOD PRESSURE

(pages 243–246 and Fig. 11.12 of Scott, Webb and Kostelnick, 5th edition)

Give a brief definition of blood pressure:

_____

_____

_____

_____

_____

_____

_____

Activity 7

Take some time to read and discuss factors that affect blood pressure listed in Box 11.4 on page 243.

List at least four factors that can affect blood pressure:

_____

_____

_____

_____

_____

Practical Exercise: Measuring Blood Pressure

Read the box 'Delegation guidelines: Measuring blood pressure' on page 244.

What do the delegation guidelines say about steps support workers need to take when taking blood pressures?

_____

_____

_____

What types of equipment do you need in order to take someone's blood pressure?

_____

_____

_____

_____

Blood Glucose Monitoring

(pages 246–247 of Scott, Webb and Kostelnick, 5th edition)

People with diabetes need to constantly monitor the level of glucose in their blood.

Why is it important for people living with diabetes to monitor their blood glucose?

_____

_____

_____

What is a normal blood glucose reading for a person not living with diabetes?

_____

_____

_____

Look at the Box on page 247 'Assessing Blood Glucose Measurements'.

List the safety and infection prevention and control steps that are important when taking a blood glucose reading.

_____

_____

_____

_____

_____

CHCAGE007:
Recognise and report risks of falls

Table of Contents

INTRODUCTION

This workbook relates to the unit CHCAGE007: Recognise and report risk of falls.

The workbook activities and final assessment tasks will enable you to:

- recognise potential risk of falls
- report the risk of falls.

To prepare for this unit and the assessment activities, we recommend that you first read Chapter 2 of Scott, Webb and Kostelnick, 5th edition, **Protecting the person and the carer**.

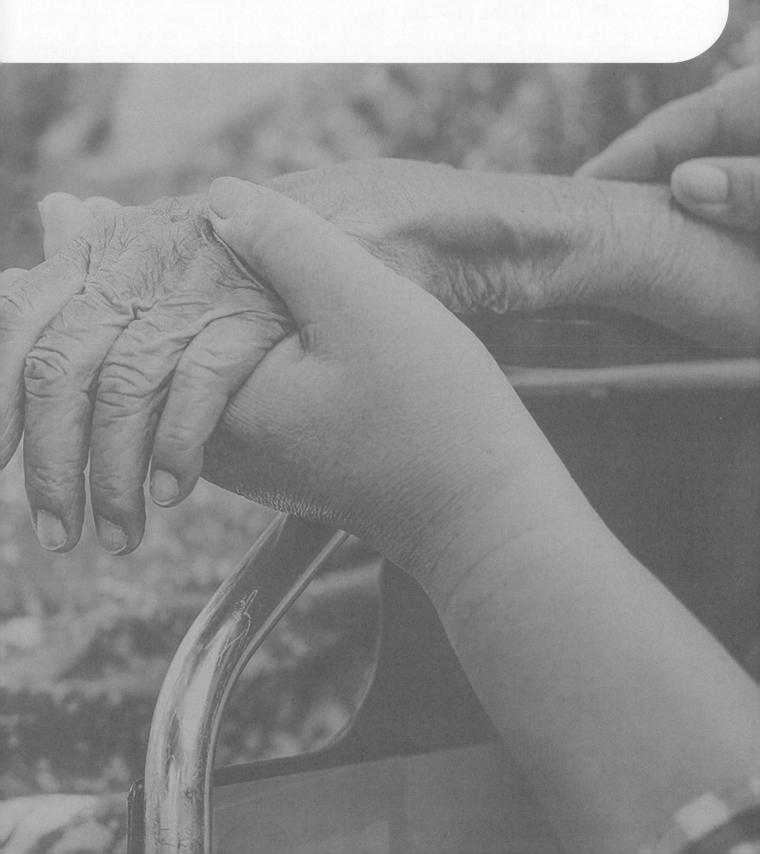

1. DEFINITION OF A FALL

(pages 28–31 of Scott, Webb and Kostelnick, 5th edition)

_____

_____

_____

_____

2. IDENTIFY POTENTIAL RISK OF FALLS

_____

_____

_____

_____

_____

3. THE AGEING PROCESS IN RELATION TO FALLS

_____

_____

_____

_____

_____

4. FACTORS CONTRIBUTING TO THE RISK OF FALLS

(Box 2.2, page 28 of Scott, Webb and Kostelnick, 5th edition)

_____

_____

_____

5. IMPACT OF FALLS ON THE PERSON AND THEIR CARER

_____

_____

_____

6. ASSESSING THE PERSON'S NORMAL GAIT AND POSTURE

_____

_____

_____

7. MEDICAL CAUSES OF FALLS AND RECOGNISING SIGNS

_____
_____
_____

8. COMMUNICATE TO PROMOTE RESPECT AND EMPOWERMENT

_____
_____
_____

9. LEGAL AND ETHICAL – DUTY OF CARE, DIGNITY OF RISK, HUMAN RIGHTS

_____
_____
_____

10. PRIVACY, CONFIDENTIALITY AND DISCLOSURE

_____
_____
_____

11. WORK, HEALTH AND SAFETY

_____
_____
_____

12. ORGANISATIONAL POLICIES AND PROCEDURES

_____
_____
_____

13. REPORT RISK OF FALLS – DOCUMENTATION AND STORAGE

(pages 6–8 of Scott, Webb and Kostelnick, 5th edition)

Refer to Boxes 2.2 and 2.3 on pages 28–29 of Scott, Webb and Kostelnick, 5th edition.

_____

_____

_____

14. RISK MANAGEMENT

(page 42 of Scott, Webb and Kostelnick, 5th edition)

Risk is defined as the possibility that an event (incident or occurrence) will occur and adversely affect the achievement of objectives.

Risk management is the practice of systematically identifying and assessing, mitigating (reducing), monitoring and reporting risks and the controls that are in place to manage and treat them.

The four steps involved in the risk management process are:

Step 1 – Identify the risk

Step 2 – Assess the risk

Step 3 – Treat/control the risk

Step 4 – Monitor effectiveness of treatment/control

Refer to Fig. 1.1 in the first Unit of this workbook.

What is a risk?

_____

_____

_____

What are the four steps in the risk management process?

_____

_____

_____

How do you report risks, accidents and incidents at your workplace?

_____

_____

_____

When undertaking a risk assessment, first you need to assess the consequence or impact of the adverse event or incident <u>before</u> you assess the likelihood of the adverse event or incident occurring.

Once the risk has been assessed, we need to implement control measures to reduce the likelihood of the adverse event occurring.

The hierarchy of control is a series of steps that should be followed to eliminate or reduce risk. The steps are listed from most effective to least effective.

How are risks identified at your workplace?

_____

_____

_____

_____

_____

_____

Activity 1

Break up into groups of two or three people. Using the table on the last page of this workbook, undertake an environmental risk assessment for falls. Think of two risks in your workplace: one physical risk (i.e. care recipient medical condition) and one environmental risk (i.e. uneven pavers). Assess the level of risk using the risk assessment matrix (see Fig. 1.2) and then work out what control measures would be suitable to eliminate or minimise the risk. Refer to the hierarchy of controls diagram (see Fig. 1.3) when working out your control measures. Record the results in the table.

Assess risks – Develop assessment criteria – Likelihood/Frequency

- Likelihood represents the number of times within a specified period in which an event or action (risk) may occur and the assessed probability of occurrence of the event or action.
- Likelihood grading levels can be expressed as frequency of occurrence:
  - **Probable** (Highly Likely to occur more than once in the next 12 months)
  - **Possible** (Likely to occur once in the next 24 months)
  - **Improbable** (Unlikely to occur once in the next 5 years)
- An important aspect to consider when estimating likelihood is the frequency and duration of exposure of employees to the risk. This can range from infrequent to continuous. Frequency of exposure is the proportion of an employee's working hours during which they are exposed to a particular risk/hazard.

Assess risks – Develop assessment criteria – Impact/Consequences

- Impact (or consequence) refers to the extent to which the occurrence of a risk event might harm an individual. Extent of harm to the individual (worker or care recipient) grading levels can be expressed as:
  - **Major** (death, major injury or illness normally resulting in long term disability).
  - **Moderate** (moderate injury or illness requiring treatment at a hospital normally resulting in short term disability).
  - **Minor** (minor injury or illness requiring treatment at the workplace with no resultant disability).

Assess risks – Develop assessment criteria – Risk Severity

- Risk severity is the risk rating derived from the aggregation of the assessed likelihood and the **highest impact** on a risk heat map. The risk severity band should be viewed from a residual risk perspective to reflect the current status of a risk (i.e. controls exist to manage inherent risks, therefore they should be considered in the overall assessment of the risk profile).
- The risk severity ratings used are based on a three-tier grading level for the **Likelihood** and **Consequence** of an identified risk (such as a Norovirus outbreak) happening. The scale used to rate each overall risk is the product (combination) of **Consequence and Likelihood** and is assessed as follows:
  - High
  - Medium
  - Low

Hierarchy of Control

Refer to Fig. 1.3 in the first Unit of this workbook.

The **Hierarchy of control** is a series of steps that should be followed to eliminate or reduce risk. The steps are listed from most effective to least effective.

1 **Eliminate** – get rid of the hazard altogether; e.g. manually lifting residents must be eliminated

2 **Substitution** – replace the hazardous practice with a less hazardous one; e.g. use a mechanical lifter or if soap is giving support workers dermatitis substitute the soap for a hypoallergenic hand wash

3 **Engineering** – ventilation system, height adjustable bed, wheels on trolley and chairs.

4 **Isolation** – store room for chemicals and locked cupboard for S8 drugs, sound proofing

5 **Administrative controls** such as policies and procedures, job rotation, training, redesigning jobs

6 **Personal Protective Equipment** (PPE) is always last as you should explore all the options above first. Also human nature dictates that people don't always wear their PPE. Examples: ear muffs, eye protection, masks, gloves

Risk	Risk Severity Rating			Control Measures (What steps we will take to reduce the risk severity rating)	Monitoring and Supervision (How compliance with the control measures will be supervised and monitored)	Person Responsible
	Likelihood	Consequence	Severity			
Physical						
Environmental						

Unit CHCCCS031:
Provide individualised support

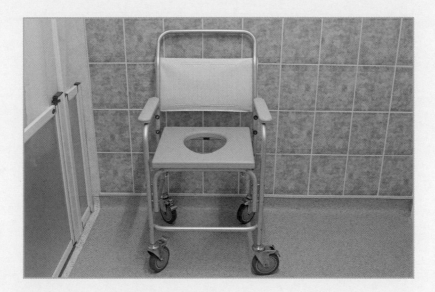

Figure 7b.1 Equipment required for personal care
(iStockphoto/shank_ali.)

Table of Contents

INTRODUCTION

This workbook relates to the unit **CHCCCS031: Provide individualised support**.

The workbook activities and final assessment tasks will enable you to:

- determine personal support requirements
- provide support services
- monitor support activities
- complete reporting and documentation.

To prepare for this unit and the assessment activities, we recommend that you first read Chapter 12 Scott, Webb and Kostelnick, 5th edition, **Caring for the person**.

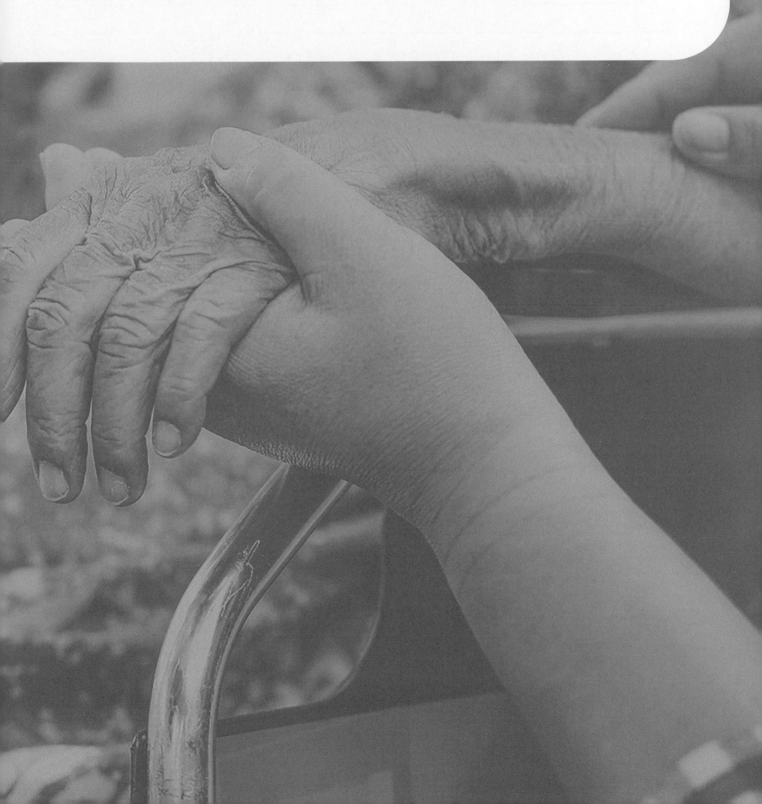

1. ASSISTING WITH HYGIENE

(pages 252–253 of Scott, Webb and Kostelnick, 5th edition)

The majority of older people remain independent throughout their lives; however, some will require help with activities of daily living, including personal care. Information about a person's hygiene needs will be found in their person-centred individualised nursing care plan. Culture and personal choice affect people's hygiene practices, and these factors will have been assessed in the planning process.

Activity 1

1 List physiological changes that affect personal hygiene needs:

_____

_____

_____

_____

_____

_____

_____

2 List resistance-to-care factors that impact personal hygiene needs:

_____

_____

_____

_____

_____

_____

_____

Activity 2

Personal hygiene will be performed daily by the client themselves or with assistance from the carer (who will work to maintain as much independence for the client as possible). In the table below, list some routine tasks that you would perform at different times of day to assist your client with their hygiene needs.

Time of day	Personal hygiene care
Morning care	
Afternoon care	
Evening care	
Oral hygiene	

(pages 253–258 of Scott, Webb and Kostelnick, 5th edition)

Oral hygiene is an important aspect of care for your older client. Why do you perform oral hygiene?

_____

_____

_____

_____

_____

Denture care

(Fig. 12.7 and pages 258–259 of Scott, Webb and Kostelnick, 5th edition)

Identify important tips in denture care.

_____

_____

_____

_____

_____

_____

_____

_____

_____

Bathing

(pages 259–269 of Scott, Webb and Kostelnick, 5th edition)

Activity 3

Mrs Crane is 93 years old with moderate dementia. She mobilises with supervision and a walking frame. She has dry skin and a skin tear on her lower left leg. Today she is going out for lunch with her daughter. As Mrs Crane's carer, outline your personal care choices as follows:

1 What bathing choice would you make for Mrs Crane?

_____

_____

_____

2 What safety considerations would you need to be aware of while delivering Mrs Crane's personal care?

_____

_____

_____

3 Describe how you would ensure that Mrs Crane's privacy and dignity are upheld during bathing and personal care.

_____

_____

_____

_____

4 Mrs Crane wants to use her 'special' talcum powder today. What would you say and do?

_____

_____

_____

5 Describe how you would prepare Mrs Crane for her lunch outing once you have assisted her to bathe, highlighting how you would maximise her independence.

_____

_____

_____

6 What would you report to the RN/supervisor after you have finished Mrs Crane's care?

_____

_____

_____

Assisting with Grooming, Skin and Nail Care

(pages 276–288 of Scott, Webb and Kostelnick, 5th edition)

Hair Care

Many older clients need the assistance of the carer to perform routine tasks associated with hair care. When planning for personal care, determine from the nursing care plan whether the client is to have their hair washed.

What do you think are three main reasons why grooming is important to clients?

_____

_____

_____

Read the shampooing guidelines on pages 277–280 of Scott, Webb and Kostelnick, 5th edition, and discuss these with your trainer and group.

Shaving

(pages 280–282 of Scott, Webb and Kostelnick, 5th edition)

Safety considerations for shaving clients:

_____

_____

_____

_____

Care of Nails and Feet

(pages 282–284 of Scott, Webb and Kostelnick, 5th edition)

Always check with facility policy. Some facilities do not allow carers to attend to the clients' toenails; these must be attended to by a podiatrist. Additionally, some facilities will not allow carers to attend to the fingernails of clients with diabetes.

What are the safety considerations for hand and nail care?

_____

_____

_____

_____

_____

_____

Read the box 'Giving nail and foot care' on page 283, and discuss the content with your trainer and group.

Dressing and Changing Clothing

(pages 284–288 of Scott, Webb and Kostelnick, 5th edition)

Activity 4

Mr Lyon is 87 years old and has a left-sided weakness following a stroke. After his shower, you proceed to assist him with dressing for the day.

1 When dressing Mr Lyon, what are the important rules to remember?

_____

_____

_____

2 How will you maximise Mr Lyon's participation while dressing him?

_____

_____

_____

2. ASSISTING WITH BOWEL EVACUATION AND MANAGEMENT

(pages 288–292 of Scott, Webb and Kostelnick, 5th edition)

Bowel evacuation is the excretion of wastes from the gastrointestinal system and is a basic physical need. There are many factors that affect bowel evacuation needs.

In the following table, give an example of ways to promote effective bowel evacuation for each of the factors listed in the first column.

Factors that affects bowel evacuation	Ways to promote effective bowel evacuation
Privacy	
Personal habits	
Diet	
Fluids	
Activity	
Medications	
Ageing	
Disability	

Activity 5

As a support worker, it is your role to document your client's defecation. Where will you record this, and what will you record?

_____

_____

_____

_____

Common problems with bowel evacuation include constipation, faecal impaction, diarrhoea and faecal incontinence. These conditions may be managed with enemas, suppositories and bowel training programs.

Read pages 290–292, and discuss these issues with your trainer and group.

3. ASSISTING WITH URINARY ELIMINATION AND MANAGEMENT

(pages 299–306 of Scott, Webb and Kostelnick, 5th edition)

Read Box 12.8 on page 300.

The urinary system removes waste products from the blood and maintains the body's water balance.

When assisting a client with urinary elimination, what important considerations must you always adhere to?

_____

_____

_____

_____

Read Box 'Helping a person to the commode' on pp. 305–306.

Activity 6

1 Where would you find information about your client's urinary elimination needs?

_____

_____

_____

2 How would you ensure your client's privacy and dignity during urinary elimination?

_____

_____

_____

3 How would you ensure you have fulfilled your duty of care for your client's safety?

_____

_____

_____

4 How would you enable your client's maximum participation?

_____

_____

_____

Urinary Incontinence

(pages 306–308 of Scott, Webb and Kostelnick, 5th edition)

Urinary incontinence is the loss of bladder control and may have multiple causes.

Read Box 12.9 on page 307, and identify issues you must observe to assist a client with urinary incontinence.

_____

_____

_____

_____

_____

_____

Urine samples are collected for testing to diagnose or to evaluate treatment. Specimens may be sent off for testing in a pathology laboratory or tested in the facility. As a carer, you may be asked to do simple urine tests using reagent strips.

Reagent strips have sections that change colour when they react with urine. To use a reagent strip, dip the strip into the urine and compare the strip to the colour chart on the bottle.

Read the box 'Testing urine with reagent strips' on page 318, and identify eight main points.

Read Box 12.12 on page 315 'Rules for collecting urine specimens'.

_____

_____

_____

_____

_____

_____

_____

4. ASSISTING WITH WOUND CARE

(pages 319–335 of Scott, Webb and Kostelnick, 5th edition)

The skin is the body's first line of defence from pathogens that may cause infection. A wound is a break in the skin or mucous membrane, and is a point of entry for pathogens.

List some common causes of skin breakdown that you are aware of.

_____

_____

_____

_____

_____

_____

_____

_____

_____

Now compare your list with that in Box 12.13 on page 319 and Box 12.17 on page 321.

One of the common types of wounds sustained by clients is a skin tear.

_____

_____

_____

Activity 7

If one of your clients should sustain a skin tear, the registered nurse/supervisor will assess the tear using the STAR classification system. The assessment outcomes will then dictate the most appropriate management of the skin tear.

Which of your clients would be most at risk of sustaining a skin tear?

_____

_____

_____

_____

What measures would you put in place to prevent skin tears?

_____

_____

_____

_____

As a carer, what would you do if you found a skin tear on one of your clients?

_____

_____

_____

_____

Pressure Injury

(pages 321–328 of Scott, Webb and Kostelnick, 5th edition)

A pressure injury is any injury caused by unrelieved pressure. It normally occurs over bony prominences.

Activity 8

On the diagrams, identify pressure points that are the most common sites for pressure injuries.

Which of your clients are most at risk of sustaining a pressure injury?

_____

_____

_____

Pressure injuries are assessed and graded according to many factors. Read Box 12.18 on page 321, then look at Figure 12.75 on page 322. Discuss the different stages of pressure injuries with your trainer and group.

Preventing pressure injuries is the main goal. Read Box 12.19 on page 324, and summarise the main points for preventing pressure injuries.

_____

_____

_____

_____

_____

_____

_____

_____

_____

_____

5. ASSISTING WITH IDENTIFYING AND MANAGING PAIN

(pages 335–338 of Scott, Webb and Kostelnick, 5th edition)

Activity 9

Pain is a personal experience. Many factors affect a person's ability to cope with pain.

Provide examples for each of the following response factors.

Factors that affect client response	Examples
Past experiences	
Anxiety	
Rest and sleep	
Reason for pain	
Support from others	
Culture	

As a carer, what is your main responsibility when your client tells you that they have pain?

_____

_____

In assessing a client's pain, you need to elicit a better picture of the pain experience. Provide examples of questions you might use in each part of the assessment process.

Assessment category	Sample question
Location	
Onset and duration	
Intensity	
Description	
Other signs and symptoms	

In a discussion with the person next to you, identify some pain-relieving measures that you both have used.

_____

_____

_____

_____

_____

_____

_____

6. ASSISTING WITH FEEDING AND DRINKING

(pages 338–342 of Scott, Webb and Kostelnick, 5th edition)

It is important to remember that eating should be enjoyed and mealtime is a pleasurable social time in a client's day.

Many factors affect a client's dietary practice. After reading pages 339–346, give examples of the following practices.

Dietary practice	Example
Culture and religion	
Ageing changes	
Social factors	
Emotional factors	
Finances	

Activity 10

It is lunchtime. Describe how you will make the mealtime as pleasurable as possible for your clients.

_____

_____

_____

_____

_____

_____

7. ASSISTING WITH EXERCISE AND ACTIVITY

(pages 356–361 of Scott, Webb and Kostelnick, 5th edition)

The Aged Care Accreditation Standard 2.14 states: 'Optimum levels of mobility and dexterity are achieved for all residents.'

Inactivity affects every body system, as well as mental wellbeing.

Each nursing care plan will inform you of how much support the client needs and how to safely prepare for each task, taking into account any risks to the client. Major goals are: encouraging exercise and activity; maintaining correct body alignment and positioning; and performing range-of-motion exercises for those who are less mobile. There are risks to each client during mobility.

One risk to the client is orthostatic hypotension. What is orthostatic hypotension?

_____

_____

_____

When getting a client out of bed, what would you do to prevent your client falling from orthostatic hypotension?

_____

_____

_____

What would you do if your client reported that they felt dizzy/faint while you were assisting them out of bed?

_____

_____

_____

Range-of-Motion (ROM) Exercises

(pages 358–361 of Scott, Webb and Kostelnick, 5th edition)

ROM exercises move the joints through their complete range of motion. The exercises may be passive (performed by the carer) or active (performed by the client). Each client is assessed by a physiotherapist, who determines the plan of care.

Assisting with ROM exercise is part of your job. What information would you need before you attend to this task?

_____

_____

_____

Walking Aids

(pages 364–368 of Scott, Webb and Kostelnick, 5th edition)

Each client will be assessed by the physiotherapist and may be advised to use a walking aid. The physiotherapist measures each person to ensure the correct size of equipment and teaches correct use of the aid.

Activity 11

For each of the walking aids shown below, name the aid, describe its correct use, and list possible risks or safety concerns.

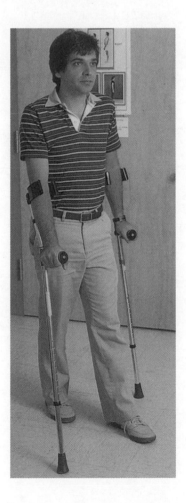

Figure 7b.2:
(Reprinted with permission from Amy M. Hall, Anne Griffin Perry, Patricia A. Potter, et al. eds. Canadian Fundamentals of Nursing, Sixth Edition. Elsevier Canada, a division of Reed Elsevier Canada, Ltd. 2019)

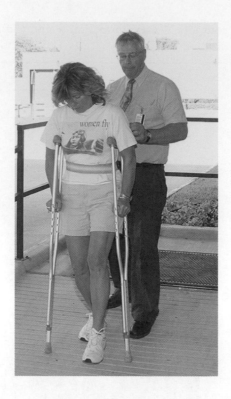

Figure 7b.3:
(Reprinted with permission from Roberta O'Shea, Sheryl Fairchild (2023). Pierson and Fairchild's Principles & Techniques of Patient Care, Seventh Edition. Elsevier Inc.)

_____

_____

_____

_____

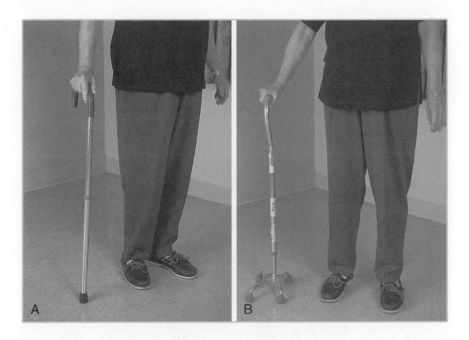

Figure 7b.4:
(Reproduced with permission from Sorrentino A & Gorek B (2011) Mosby's textbook for long-term care nursing assistants (6th edn), Mosby, St Louis)

_____

_____

_____

_____

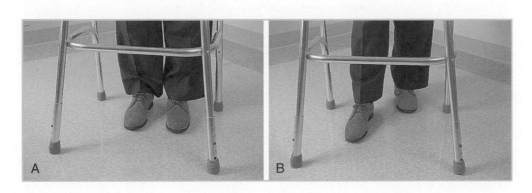

Figure 7b.5:
(Reproduced with permission from Sorrentino A & Gorek B (2003) Mosby's textbook for long-term care assistants (4th edn), Mosby, St Louis)

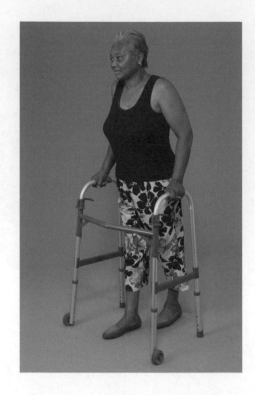

Figure 7b.6:
(Reprinted with permission from Sheila A. Sorrentino, Leighann N. Remmert (2017). Mosby's Textbook for Nursing Assistants, Ninth Edition. Elsevier Inc.)

_____

_____

_____

_____

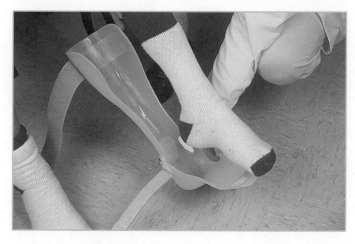

Figure 7b.7:
(Reproduced with permission from Sorrentino A & Gorek B (2011) Mosby's textbook for long-term care nursing assistants (6th edn), Mosby, St Louis)

_____

_____

_____

_____

The Falling Person

(pages 362–364 of Scott, Webb and Kostelnick, 5th edition)

Name the most important safety issue for both you and the client if your client starts to fall.

_____

_____

_____

You have a duty of care to your client. List the steps you would take if your client has a fall.

_____

_____

_____

_____

Unit CHCCCS040:
Support independence and wellbeing

Table of Contents

INTRODUCTION

This workbook relates to the unit **CHCCCS040: Support independence and wellbeing**.

The workbook activities and final assessment tasks will enable you to:

- recognise and support individual differences
- promote independence
- support physical wellbeing
- support social, emotional and psychological wellbeing.

To prepare for this unit and the assessment activities, we recommend that you first read Chapter 5 of Scott, Webb and Kostelnick, 5th edition, **Working in Home and Community Sector**.

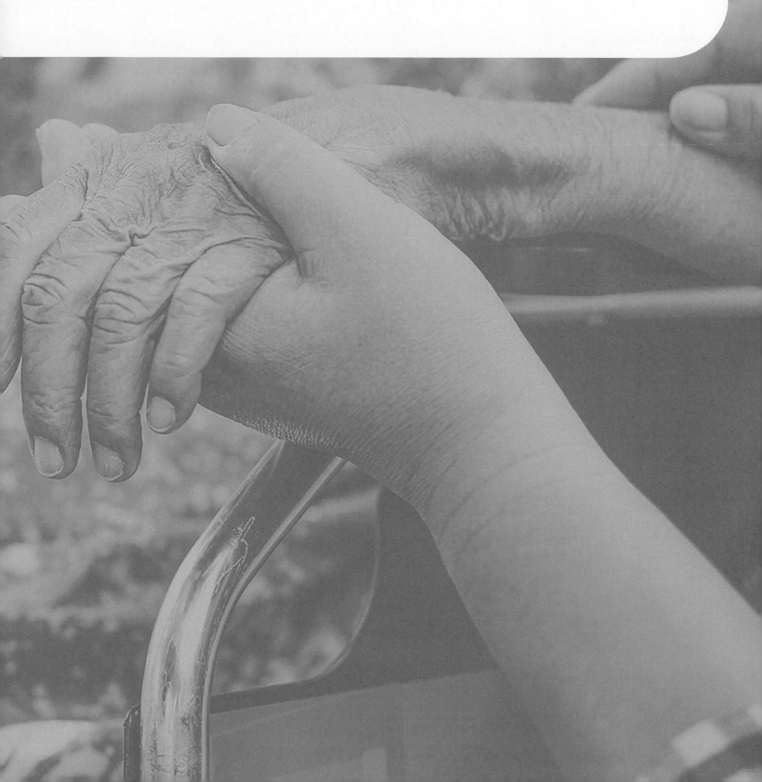

1. SERVICE DELIVERY MODELS AND STANDARDS

(pages 116–118 of Scott, Webb and Kostelnick, 5th edition)

Most older people prefer to maintain their independence and live in their own home. There are various service delivery models available for home and residential aged care.

Home Care Packages to assist people to live independently in their own home:

_____

_____

_____

_____

Residential aged care:

_____

_____

_____

_____

Funding models for home care packages for people living at home:

_____

_____

_____

_____

Funding models for people living in residential aged care:

_____

_____

_____

_____

Needs

Read pages 123, 125 and 170–171 of Scott, Webb and Kostelnick, 5th edition

All humans have basic needs that are important for their health and wellbeing:

Physical needs

_____

_____

Psychological needs

_____

_____

Spiritual needs

_____

_____

Cultural needs

_____

_____

Sexual needs

_____

_____

Social needs

_____

_____

Financial needs

_____

_____

Career/occupation needs

_____

_____

Issues that impact health and wellbeing:

_____

_____

_____

_____

2. ATTITUDES, STEREOTYPES AND MYTHS ASSOCIATED WITH AGEING

Cultural Awareness and Cultural Senstivity

(page 156 of Scott, Webb and Kostelnick, 5th edition)

List some attitudes, stereotypes and myths associated with ageing.

_____

_____

_____

_____

Elder Abuse

(page 87 of Scott, Webb and Kostelnick, 5th edition)

Read Box 3.1 on page 88.

Elder abuse is an issue that can impact on a person's health and wellbeing. What are some indicators that an older person might be subject to neglect and/or elder abuse?

_____

_____

_____

_____

If you suspect an older person is being abused, what reporting requirements are in place?

_____

_____

_____

_____

Restrictive Practices

(pages 85–86 Scott, Webb and Kostelnick, 5th edition)

From 1 July 2021, approved aged care providers have specific responsibilities under the *Aged Care Act 1997* and the Quality of Care Principles 2014 relating to the use of any restrictive practice in a residential aged care setting.

_____

_____

_____

_____

_____

_____

3. LEGAL AND ETHICAL REQUIREMENTS

(page 89–93 of Scott, Webb and Kostelnick, 5th edition)

When working in aged care there are certain legal and ethical requirements you need to abide by:

Duty of care:

_____

_____

Dignity of risk:

_____

_____

Human rights:

_____

_____

Laws against discrimination:

_____

_____

Mandatory reporting:

_____

_____

Privacy, confidentiality and disclosure:

_____

_____

Work role boundaries – responsibilities and limitations:

_____

_____

4. NUTRITION AND HYDRATION

(pages 339–343 and 371–375 of Scott, Webb and Kostelnick, 5th edition)

_____

_____

_____

_____

_____

5. DIET

Read Box 13.1 on page 371.

Activity 1

Mrs Black lives at home. She is overweight and has osteoarthritis in her hips and knees. Mrs Black doesn't exercise, as she says it causes her pain. She does her food shopping online for delivery by the supermarket, and often eats more refined carbohydrates, such as chocolate and cakes. Mrs Black thinks that drinking tea and coffee means her fluid intake is adequate. What suggestions could you make to Mrs Black to ensure that she eats a balanced diet, gets adequate hydration and is able to do some exercise each day? How could you assist her with this change?

_____

_____

_____

_____

_____

_____

_____

_____

_____

_____

_____

6. CHANGES TO NUTRITION AND HYDRATION DUE TO AGEING

(pages 371–372 of Scott, Webb and Kostelnick, 5th edition)

_____

_____

_____

_____

Loss of taste:

_____

_____

_____

_____

Ill-fitting dentures:

_____

_____

_____

_____

Decreased secretion of stomach acid:

_____

_____

_____

_____

7. THE AUSTRALIAN GUIDE TO HEALTHY EATING

Read about the Australian Guide to Healthy Eating on page 372.

_____

_____

_____

_____

_____

_____

_____

8. THE AUSTRALIAN GUIDE TO HEALTHY EATING FOR VEGETARIANS AND VEGANS

_____

_____

_____

_____

_____

9. RECREATIONAL ACTIVITIES

(pages 375–376 of Scott, Webb and Kostelnick, 5th edition)

The benefits of recreational activities for the older adult include:

_____

_____

_____

_____

_____

10. FITNESS

Read Box 13.3 on page 376.

_____

_____

_____

_____

_____

_____

_____

_____

_____

11. BODY WORK

(page 375–379 of Scott, Webb and Kostelnick, 5th edition)

Read Box 13.4 on page 376.

Massage

_____

_____

_____

_____

Benefits of massage

_____

_____

_____

_____

12. COMPLEMENTARY THERAPIES

_____
_____
_____
_____
_____

13. COMFORT, REST AND SLEEP

_____
_____
_____
_____

Activity 2

The Aged Care Accreditation Standards lists some points on how to provide a safe and comfortable environment.
Give two examples of how you can achieve comfort for the person.

_____
_____
_____
_____
_____
_____
_____
_____
_____
_____

Factors that can affect a person's sleep include:

_____
_____
_____
_____
_____

14. PROMOTING SLEEP

(pages 381 of Scott, Webb and Kostelnick, 5th edition)

Read Box 13.7 on page 381 and discuss with the class.

15. GOOD HEALTH

Oral health

_____

_____

_____

_____

_____

Hygiene

_____

_____

_____

_____

_____

Assisting with exercise and activity

_____

_____

_____

_____

_____

Mental health

_____

_____

_____

_____

_____

16. SPIRITUAL, CULTURAL AND SEXUAL NEEDS OF THE PERSON

(page 125 of Scott, Webb and Kostelnick, 5th edition)

In your role as carer, whether it be in the residential aged care setting or community setting, how do you recognise and respect the person's social, cultural and spiritual differences?

_____

_____

_____

_____

_____

How could you facilitate opportunities for the person you are caring for to participate in activities that reflects the person's individual preferences?

_____

_____

_____

_____

_____

_____

_____

_____

Lesbian, Gay, Bisexual, Transgender and Intersex (LGBTIQA)

The Australian Institute of Family Studies (2019) sets out in its resource sheet a glossary of terms relating to LGBTIQA.

1 _____

2 _____

3 _____

4 _____

5 _____

6 _____

7 _____

Take some time to discuss with your trainer and the group how you could implement these goals into your care.

Unit CHCAGE011:
Provide support to people living with dementia

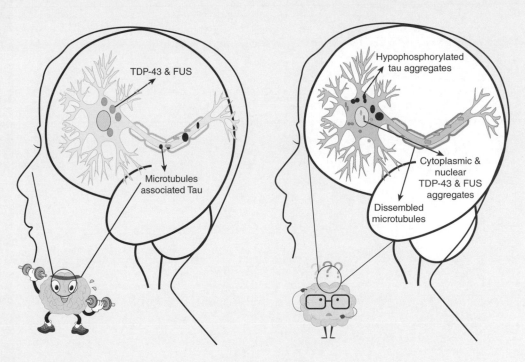

Figure 9.1 **Aetiopathogenesis of frontotemporal dementia.**
(Reprinted with permission from Nanomedicine-Based Approaches for the Treatment of Dementia, First Edition. Elsevier Inc. 2023.)

Table of Contents

INTRODUCTION

This workbook relates to the unit **CHCAGE011 Provide support to people living with dementia** and **CHCCS044 Follow established person-centred behaviour supports**.

The workbook activities and final assessment tasks will enable you to:

- prepare to provide support to those affected by dementia
- use effective communication strategies
- support the person to participate in activities according to individualised plan
- use a strengths-based approach to meet the person's needs
- complete documentation
- apply a person-centred approach to providing behaviour support
- review context of behaviours of concern
- provide positive behaviour support according to individualised behaviour support plans

To prepare for this unit and the assessment activities, we recommend that you first read Chapter 14 of Scott, Webb and Kostelnick, 5th edition, **Working with people living with dementia**.

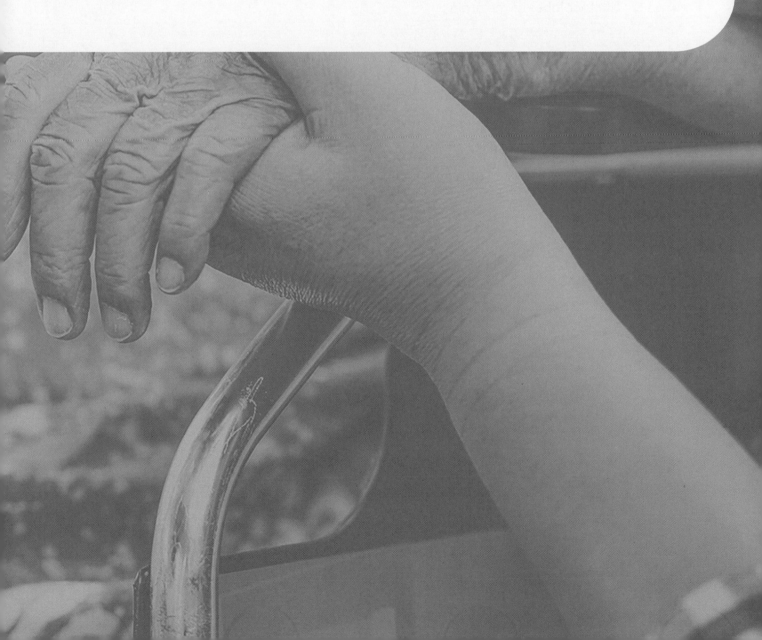

1. THE BRAIN

(page 387 of Scott, Webb and Kostelnick, 5th edition)

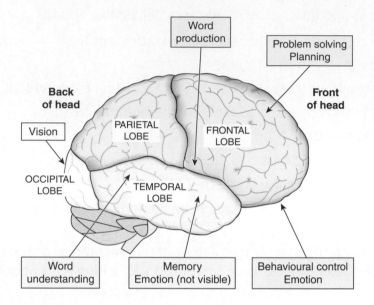

Figure 9.2 The four lobes of the brain.

Activity 1

The brain has four main lobes. Describe the changes to each lobe when damaged.

1 Frontal lobe:

_____

_____

2 Parietal lobe:

_____

_____

3 Temporal lobe:

_____

_____

4 Occipital lobe:

_____

_____

Cognitive Function

(page 387 of Scott, Webb and Kostelnick, 5th edition)

Describe cognitive function:

_____

_____

_____

_____

_____

_____

_____

_____

_____

_____

_____

2. CONFUSION

(pages 387–388 of Scott, Webb and Kostelnick, 5th edition)

Read Box 14.2 on page 388, Caring for the confused person.

Confusion has many causes and is often reversible. List the main causes of confusion:

_____

_____

_____

_____

_____

_____

_____

_____

_____

3. DELIRIUM

(pages 388–389 of Scott, Webb and Kostelnick, 5th edition)

_____

_____

What are the signs and symptoms of delirium?

_____

_____

_____

_____

_____

Depression

(pages 389 of Scott, Webb and Kostelnick, 5th edition)

_____

_____

_____

_____

Depression is the most common mental health problem in older people and is often confused with dementia. A correct diagnosis is needed for proper treatment. List the signs and symptoms of depression.

_____

_____

_____

_____

_____

_____

4. DEMENTIA

(pages 389–390 of Scott, Webb and Kostelnick, 5th edition)

Dementia is not a normal part of ageing. If you had to describe dementia to a relative, what would you say?

_____

_____

_____

_____

_____

_____

Identify three early warning signs of dementia.

_____

_____

_____

_____

Overview of dementia types:.

(pages 390–392 of Scott, Webb and Kostelnick, 5th edition)

_____

_____

_____

_____

_____

_____

_____

_____

_____

_____

_____

_____

5. ALZHEIMER'S DISEASE

(pages 392–394 of Scott, Webb and Kostelnick, 5th edition)

Alzheimer's disease is the most common form of dementia. It causes a gradual decline in cognitive abilities, with the family first noticing short-term memory loss. Alzheimer's disease is characterised by two abnormalities in the brain – amyloid plaques and neuro-fibrillary tangles. These plaques and tangles stop communication between nerve cells and cause the cell to die.

Activity 2

List signs and symptoms of Alzheimer's disease. Classify them as either a care issue or a safety issue.

Care issue	Safety issue

Stages of Dementia

(page 395–396 of Scott, Webb and Kostelnick, 5th edition)

Each person goes through the journey of dementia at an individual pace, but symptoms do become more severe as each stage progresses. Alzheimer's disease is progressive and irreversible.

Read Box 14.1. As a group, discuss the needs of a person living with dementia disease as they move through each stage. Use the headings below as a discussion guide.

Personal care needs	Safety and security needs
Nutrition needs	Social/Leisure needs
Communication needs	Mobility needs
Need for a stable and familiar environment	

Behavioural and Psychological Symptoms of Dementia (BPSD)

(pages 394–395 and 398 of Scott, Webb and Kostelnick, 5th edition)

People with dementia may exhibit many changed behaviours as a result of their condition.

Activity 3

For each of these behaviours, provide a definition and a strategy for managing the behaviour.

1 Wandering:

_____

_____

_____

2 Hallucinations:

_____

_____

_____

3 Delusions:

_____

_____

_____

4 Agitation and restlessness:

_____

_____

_____

5 Aggression and combativeness:

_____

_____

_____

6 Screaming:

_____

_____

_____

7 Abnormal sexual behaviours:

_____

_____

_____

8 Repetitive behaviour:

_____

_____

_____

9 Sundowning:

_____

_____

_____

10 Catastrophic reactions:

_____

_____

_____

Changed Behaviours

(pages 394 and 401 of Scott, Webb and Kostelnick, 5th edition)

People with dementia cannot control what is happening to them. If you try to determine what is triggering the changed behaviour, you may be able to prevent it from recurring. Think ABC.

A_____

B_____

C_____

Activity 4: Case study

It is dinnertime in your facility and Kev, a new care recipient, has finished his meal. He reaches across the table and takes Matt's dessert. Matt hits out at Kev. There is shouting and commotion. An inexperienced care worker rushes over and raises her voice at Matt, who then pushes his teacup to the floor.

Using the ABC tool for Kev complete the table.

	For Kev
Antecedent	
Behaviour	
Consequence	

1. How should the support worker have handled the situation?

_____

_____

_____

_____

2. What systems could be put in place to prevent this from happening again?

_____

_____

_____

_____

3. Management of behaviours depends on triggers. Once we have identified the triggers we can put strategies into place to minimise the behaviour. What strategies can you put into place to minimise changed behaviours?

_____

_____

_____

_____

_____

_____

_____

_____

6. CARE OF THE PERSON WITH DEMENTIA

(pages 396–400 of Scott, Webb and Kostelnick, 5th edition)

Activity 5

People with dementia who exhibit changed behaviours often do so due to unmet needs.

Look at the following list of support needs, and identify some strategies that you can implement to meet these needs.

Safety:

_____

_____

_____

Hygiene:

_____

_____

_____

Nutrition:

_____

_____

_____

Fluids:

_____

_____

_____

Elimination:

_____

_____

_____

_____

_____

Comfort:

_____

_____

_____

Sleep:

_____

_____

_____

Dignity and respect:

_____

_____

_____

Elder Abuse

Elder abuse is a pattern of behaviour that causes physical, psychological, financial or social harm to an older person. Support workers owe a duty of care to clients to keep them safe. People living with dementia are more likely to be abused, as they cannot always speak up about the abuse and so it may go undetected.

Abuse may be physical, psychological, financial, sexual, exploitation or as a result of neglect. Abuse may be carried out by partners, friends, family members, support workers, carers or health professionals. Abuse can occur at home or in a residential aged care setting.

Activity 6

For each type of abuse, list some indications for that abuse.

Type of abuse	Indications of abuse
Physical	
Psychological	
Financial	
Sexual	
Exploitation	
Neglect	

Communication (Verbal and Non-Verbal)

(pages 399–400 of Scott, Webb and Kostelnick, 5th edition)

'Communication is made up of three parts:

- 55% body language, facial expression posture and gestures
- 38% tone and pitch of our voice
- 7% the words we use.' (www.alzheimers.org.au)

The person who is having difficulty communicating may pick up on negative body language such as crossed arms and eye rolling. When communicating with the care recipient, always maintain their dignity and self-esteem. Allow time for a response from the person. Use touch to keep the person's attention and to communicate feelings of warmth.

List some verbal and non-verbal communication strategies you can use with someone living with dementia:

_____

_____

_____

_____

_____

_____

Activity 7

In 1995, Christine Bryden (Boden) was diagnosed with dementia at age 46. She has written a book called *Who Will I Be When I Die?* Imagine you are a person with dementia. What suggestions could you give to people on how to communicate with you effectively?

_____

_____

_____

_____

_____

_____

_____

_____

_____

_____

Other Communication Strategies

(pages 399–400 of Scott, Webb and Kostelnick, 5th edition)

Activity 8

From your experience of dealing with people with dementia, give some examples of each of the following strategies.

Reminiscence: Remembering and reflecting on previous life events and experiences.

_____

_____

_____

Redirection: Redirection of thoughts to something that is more pleasant.

_____

_____

_____

Validation: Entering the person's reality; recognising the person's thoughts and emotions.

_____

_____

_____

Reality orientation: Orientating the person to time and place.

_____

_____

_____

Music therapy: An enjoyable experience which can unlock memories and feelings.

_____

_____

_____

Using sense of smell: Smell can trigger powerful memories.

_____

_____

_____

Complete Documentation

Documentation is a term used for any written information that an organisation collects. Aged care organisations use documentation for the following purposes:

_____

_____

_____

_____

_____

_____

Reporting gives an oral account of care and observations. *Recording* means writing an account of care and observations.

Activity 9

What are some types of reporting and documentation required from you as a support worker in your organisation?

_____

_____

_____

_____

_____

Caregivers

(page 401–402 of Scott, Webb and Kostelnick, 5th edition)

The person with dementia may live at home with family members or in a residential aged care facility. As a family member giving care, there can be positive and negative aspects of being a caregiver.

Positive aspects of being a caregiver:

_____

_____

_____

_____

Negative aspects of being a caregiver:

_____

_____

_____

_____

_____

_____

Carer Stress and Self-Care

Working with people with dementia can be stressful. You take on the dual role of caring for the person with dementia as well as their relatives. It is important that you monitor your own stress level in relation to your work.

Activity 10

1 Signs and symptoms that your body is under stress:

_____

_____

_____

_____

_____

_____

_____

2 Healthy strategies to help you cope with stress:

_____

_____

_____

_____

_____

_____

10

Unit CHCPAL003:
Deliver care services using a palliative approach

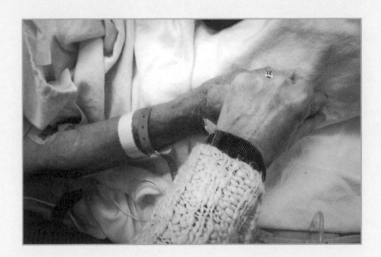

Figure 10.1 Hospice care
(iStockphoto/-Oxford-.)

Table of Contents

INTRODUCTION

This workbook relates to the unit **CHCPAL003: Deliver care services using a palliative approach** and **CHCCCS017 Provide loss and grief support**.

The workbook activities and final assessment tasks will enable you to:

- apply principles and aims of a palliative approach when supporting people
- respect the person's preferences for quality-of-life choices
- follow the person's advance care directives in the individualised plan
- respond to signs of pain and other symptoms
- follow end-of-life care strategies
- manage own emotional responses and ethical issues.
- recognise reactions to loss and grief
- engage empathically
- offer support and information
- care for self
- review support provided.

To prepare for this unit and the assessment activities, we recommend that you first read Chapter 17 of Scott, Webb and Kostelnick, 5th edition, **Working with older clients requiring palliative care**.

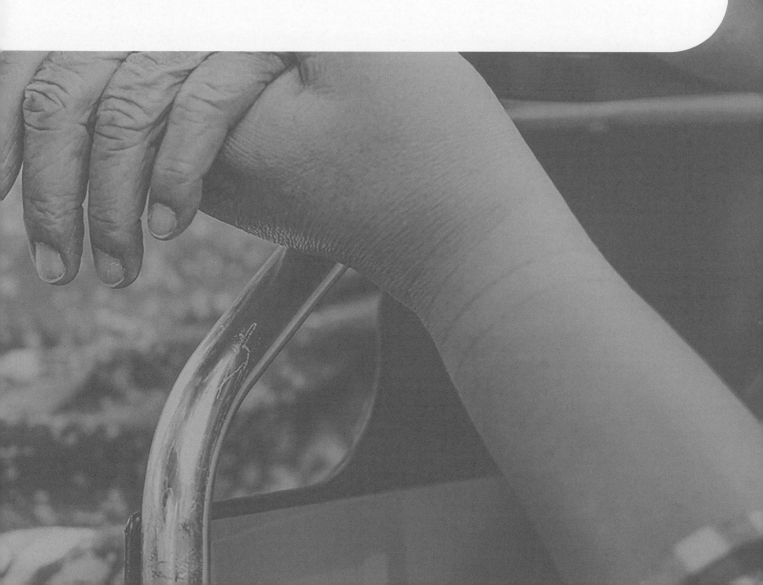

1. LOSS AND GRIEF

(page 429 of Scott, Webb and Kostelnick, 5th edition)

Loss, grief, death and dying are all part of the life cycle.

Describe loss:

_____

_____

_____

_____

_____

Describe grief:

_____

_____

_____

_____

Responses to loss and grief are personal. Can you think of types of losses that an aged person and their family may experience?

Types of loss	Examples of responses

Responses to grief may be influenced by cultural, religious and spiritual beliefs. As a carer, you will encounter clients and families responding to grief in many ways. Responses may include:

Emotional responses:

_____

_____

_____

Physical responses:

_____

_____

_____

Cognitive responses:

_____

_____

_____

_____

2. ATTITUDES TO DEATH AND DYING

(page 429 of Scott, Webb and Kostelnick, 5th edition)

People hold many different beliefs and attitudes about death and dying. After reading the text, list some of these attitudes.

_____

_____

_____

_____

_____

_____

_____

_____

_____

3. STAGES OF GRIEF

(page 430 of Scott, Webb and Kostelnick, 5th edition)

Dr Elisabeth Kubler-Ross identified five stages of grief in her text _On Death and Dying_ (1969). After reading about these in your text, summarise the five stages.

1 Denial:

_____

_____

_____

2 Anger:

_____

_____

_____

3 Bargaining:

_____

_____

_____

4 Depression:

_____

_____

_____

5 Acceptance:

_____

_____

_____

Do you think all people move through all these five stages before they die?

_____

_____

_____

_____

_____

4. CULTURE, RELIGION AND DEATH RITES

(pages 430–431 of Scott, Webb and Kostelnick, 5th edition)

After reading your text, choose one of the cultures mentioned and write about their unique death rites.

_____

_____

_____

_____

_____

_____

_____

5. PALLIATIVE CARE

(pages 431–434 of Scott, Webb and Kostelnick, 5th edition)

What do you think the term 'palliative care' means?

_____

_____

_____

_____

_____

Describe the aims of palliative care:

_____

_____

_____

_____

Define the following terms:

Curative care:

_____

_____

_____

Terminal illness:

_____

_____

Palliative care team:

_____

_____

Advance care directive:

_____

_____

_____

_____

_____

_____

_____

Palliative Care Team

A team approach to care planning facilitates provision of holistic care. Name some of the members of the palliative care team (multidisciplinary team).

_____

_____

_____

_____

_____

_____

_____

_____

6. PALLIATIVE CARE OF THE INDIVIDUAL

(pages 431–434 of Scott, Webb and Kostelnick, 5th edition)

Activity 1

The overall aim of palliative care is to promote physical, psychological, emotional and spiritual support for the individual. For each of these physical and sensory care needs, identify a strategy to manage the need:

Care need	Management strategy
Skin care	
Personal hygiene	
Oral hygiene	
Mobility and positioning	
Pain management	
Urinary continence	
Bowel elimination	
Body temperature	
Swallowing difficulty (dysphagia)	
Breathing difficulty (dyspnoea)	
Vision impairment	
Communication deficit	
Nutrition and hydration	

Pain

One of the main aims of palliative care is relief from pain. Pain is subjective; therefore, each person will experience pain individually. How would you describe pain?

_____

_____

_____

_____

Activity 2

Pain management is dependent on impeccable pain assessment. Pain can be managed with medication and non-medication strategies. List some of these.

Medication strategies	Non-medication strategies

Advance Care Planning

Advance care planning is a process to help the client plan their care in advance so that, if they become too unwell to make decisions for themselves, their wishes can still be respected by the healthcare team, family and carers.

Activity 3

Imagine you became very sick and couldn't communicate to your healthcare team about your treatment. What would you want in your advance care plan that would determine the type and level of medical intervention to be undertaken?

This might include:

- types of treatment you would or would not accept
- specific conditions that you would find unacceptable
- who you would appoint as your enduring guardian
- any non-medical aspects of care that are important to you – for example, where you might choose to die or possible organ donation.

Draft your thoughts for your own advance care plan.

_____

_____

_____

_____

_____

_____

_____

7. PSYCHOLOGICAL, SOCIAL AND SPIRITUAL COMFORT

(pages 433–434 of Scott, Webb and Kostelnick, 5th edition)

Communication skills

There are two main communication skills that you use while caring for someone in a palliative care environment: active listening and therapeutic touch. Give some examples of how you can use these skills.

Active listening:

_____

_____

_____

Therapeutic touch:

_____

_____

_____

Activity 4

1. Spiritual needs

Name some ways you can be sensitive to the spiritual needs of your client.

_____

_____

_____

_____

2. The person's room

A client may have palliative care delivered at home, or in an aged care facility, hospital or hospice. Describe how you would set up and maintain a person's room, and the role the family might play.

_____

_____

_____

_____

_____

8. SIGNS OF DEATH

(page 434 of Scott, Webb and Kostelnick, 5th edition)

As a person approaches death, the carer should be aware of orders relating to the client so that they do not perform procedures that are not in accordance with the care plan. Common signs and symptoms that death may be imminent may include:

_____

_____

_____

_____

_____

9. WHEN DEATH OCCURS

Describe what steps need to be taken when death occurs.

_____

_____

_____

_____

10. CARE OF THE BODY AFTER DEATH

(pages 435–436 of Scott, Webb and Kostelnick, 5th edition)

The carer may be required to perform post-mortem care. This care is performed to maintain good appearance of the body. Always refer to your facility's policies and procedures.

_____

_____

_____

_____

_____
_____
_____
_____

Carer Emotional Response

If you are overwhelmed by negative emotions after the death of a client, what would be some positive actions you could take to deal with these emotions?

_____
_____
_____
_____
_____

11. ETHICAL PRINCIPLES FOR PALLIATIVE CARE

At all times, carers should maintain the highest standards of palliative care, and ethical and moral standards. If you are asked by a client, family or care team member to perform a task you are not comfortable with, check your facility's code of ethics or consult with your supervisor.

Activity 5

Give an example of a situation where you faced an ethical dilemma when caring for someone receiving palliative care and how you dealt with this situation.

_____
_____
_____
_____
_____
_____
_____

11

Unit HLTHPS006:
Assist clients with medication

Written by Penny Kraemer

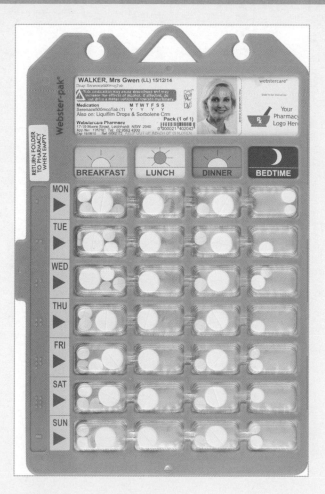

Figure 11.1 Webster-Pak® – dose administration aid
(Courtesy of Webster-pak)

Table of Contents

INTRODUCTION

This workbook relates to the unit **HLTHPS006: Assist clients with medication**.

The workbook activities and final assessment tasks will enable you to:

- prepare to assist with medication
- prepare the client for assistance with administration of medication
- support clients with administration of medication
- handle medication contingencies
- complete medication distribution.

To prepare for this unit and the assessment activities, we recommend that you first read the following chapters of Scott, Webb and Kostelnick, 5th edition: Chapter 18 on **Medications** and Chapter 1 on **Health and aged care services in Australia and New Zealand**, which sets out delegation guidelines.

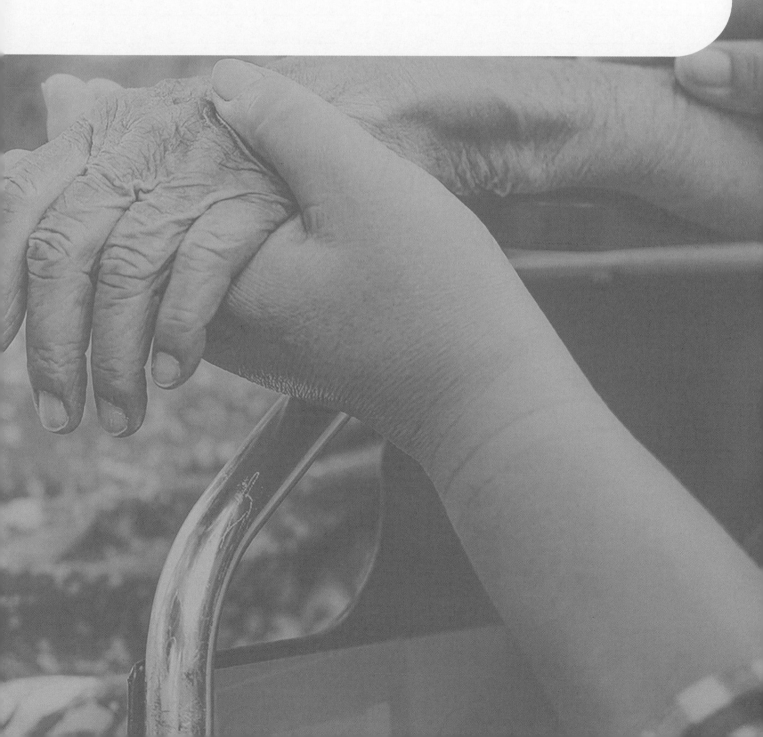

1. WHAT ARE MEDICATIONS?
(page 441 of Scott, Webb and Kostelnick, 5th edition)

_____

_____

_____

_____

_____

_____

_____

_____

2. GENERIC BRANDS OF MEDICATIONS

_____

_____

_____

_____

_____

_____

_____

_____

_____

_____

_____

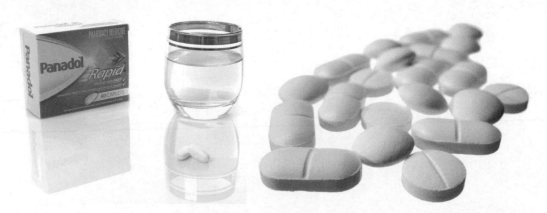

Figure 11.2 Paracetamol (generic name): Different trade names, Panadol, Herron, Coles, Dymadon
(istockphoto/lovleah (panadol box) istockphoto/stockcam (pills))

3. EFFECTS OF MEDICATION ON OLDER PEOPLE

(page 441 of Scott, Webb and Kostelnick, 5th edition)

_____
_____
_____
_____
_____
_____
_____
_____
_____
_____
_____

4. POLYPHARMACY

Describe polypharmacy.

_____
_____
_____
_____
_____
_____

5. MEDICATION ASSISTANCE

(page 441 of Scott, Webb and Kostelnick, 5th edition)

Prepare to assist with medication:

_____
_____
_____
_____
_____
_____
_____
_____
_____
_____
_____

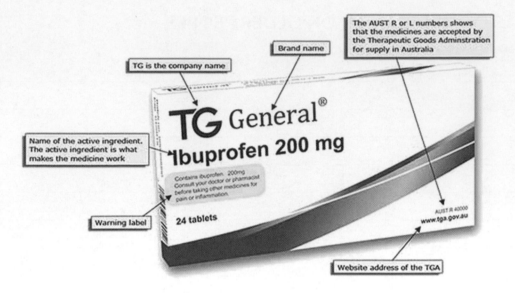

Figure 11.3 Medication instructions
(TGA medicine labelling and packaging review, 2012, Therapeutic Goods Administration, used by permission of the Australian Government, www.tga.gov.au/book/export/html/1942)

Prepare the client for assistance with administration of medication:

_____

_____

_____

_____

_____

_____

_____

Equipment Required for Medication Assistance

(page 447 of Scott, Webb and Kostelnick, 5th edition)

Look at Table 18.1 and spend some time discussing the equipment required for medication assistance.

_____

_____

_____

_____

_____

6. SUPPORTING CLIENTS WITH ADMINISTRATION OF MEDICATION

Rights of medication administration

(page 442 of Scott, Webb and Kostelnick, 5th edition)

See Box 18.2 on page 442. When you give someone their medications, you must ensure that you adhere to the seven rights of medication administration. List them here.

1 _____

2 _____

3 _____

4 _____

5 _____

6 _____

7 _____

Activity 1

You are assisting with medications. The person says to you, 'I saw the doctor and I usually take two of these green tablets, not one.' Do you give the person two or one? How would you go about finding out what dose the person should be taking, and what do you say to the resident?

_____

_____

_____

_____

_____

_____

_____

_____

_____

_____

_____

_____

_____

7. SELF-ADMINISTRATION OF MEDICATION

(page 442 of Scott, Webb and Kostelnick, 5th edition)

Activity 2

Someone might take their medication independently, but ask you a question such as, 'Why is this tablet a different shape or colour from my normal tablet?' List some possible explanations for why the tablet is different. What risks can you identify? How would you respond to the person?

_____

_____

_____

_____

_____

_____

_____

_____

_____

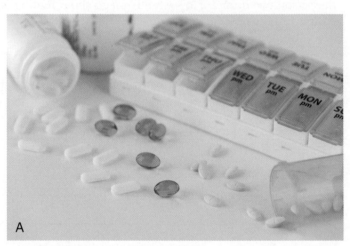

Figure 11.4 Pill organisers
(A: iStockphoto/LeeAnnWhite; B: iStockphoto/stockcam.)

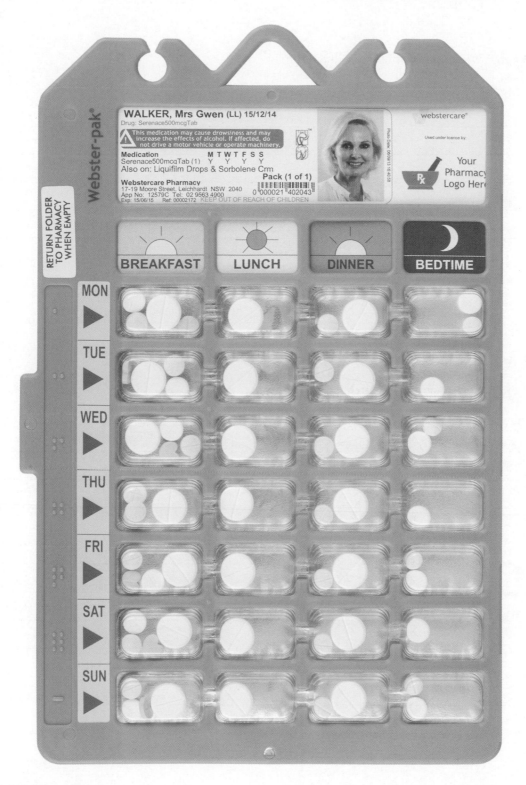

Figure 11.5 Webster-Pak®
(Courtesy of Webster-pak)

8. LEGISLATION

(pages 443 of Scott, Webb and Kostelnick, 5th edition)

Commonwealth and state regulations

_____

_____

_____

_____

_____

_____

_____

_____

9. DELEGATION

(pages 443–444 of Scott, Webb and Kostelnick, 5th edition)

_____

_____

_____

_____

_____

_____

_____

_____

_____

_____

_____

_____

_____

_____

_____

_____

_____

_____

8. LEGISLATION

(pages 443 of Scott, Webb and Kostelnick, 5th edition)

Activity 3

You completed your medication training as part of your Certificate IV in Aged Care four years ago. You have had two children and have had a three-year break from working. You have just returned to the residential aged care facility and are working in low care. You are still trying to familiarise yourself with all the residents. The registered nurse (RN) asks you to assist with the medication administration and you don't feel confident to undertake the task.

Think back to the section on 'Refusing a task' on page 444 of Scott, Webb and Kostelnick, 5th edition. How could you let the RN know that you don't feel confident to undertake the task of assisting with medication administration? Write a half-page note to the RN, and include examples of why you don't feel you should be undertaking this task.

_____
_____
_____
_____
_____
_____
_____
_____
_____

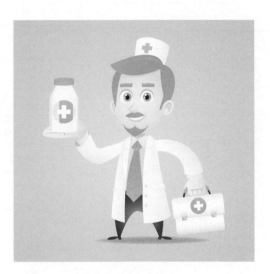

Figure 11.6 **The nurse's role includes administering medications**
(iStockphoto/Yuriy Tsirkunov.)

10. INFECTION CONTROL

Preventing contamination of aids used to apply medication.

---

11. MAINTAINING A MEDICATION RECORD

(page 444 of Scott, Webb and Kostelnick, 5th edition)

_____
_____
_____
_____
_____
_____
_____
_____
_____
_____
_____
_____
_____
_____
_____
_____
_____

12. MEDICATION INCIDENT REPORTING

(page 445 of Scott, Webb and Kostelnick, 5th edition)

_____
_____
_____
_____
_____
_____
_____
_____
_____
_____
_____
_____
_____
_____

Activity 4

1 Failure to report a medication incident can have serious consequences for the client. What could happen to the client if you failed to report a medication incident?

_____

_____

_____

_____

_____

_____

2 What could happen to you as a care worker if you fail to report a medication incident?

_____

_____

_____

_____

_____

13. ELECTRONIC MEDICATION MANAGEMENT SYSTEM (EMMS)

(pages 444–445 of Scott, Webb and Kostelnick, 5th edition)

_____

_____

_____

14. STORING MEDICATIONS

(page 445 of Scott, Webb and Kostelnick, 5th edition)

_____

_____

_____

_____

_____

_____

_____

_____

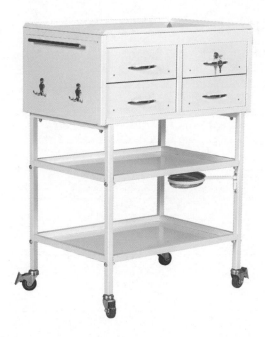

Figure 11.7 Medication trolley
(Shutterstock/Maffi.)

15. ROUTES OF ADMINISTRATION OF MEDICATIONS

(page 445 of Scott, Webb and Kostelnick, 5th edition)

Read Box 18.4 on page 445.

_____

_____

_____

_____

_____

_____

_____

_____

_____

_____

_____

_____

_____

_____

_____

16. TYPES OF MEDICATIONS

(pages 445–446 of Scott, Webb and Kostelnick, 5th edition)

_____

_____

_____

_____

_____

_____

_____

_____

_____

_____

_____

_____

17. OBSERVING FOR CHANGES IN A CLIENT'S CONDITION AFTER MEDICATION INTAKE

(page 449 of Scott, Webb and Kostelnick, 5th edition)

_____

_____

_____

_____

_____

_____

_____

Activity 5

In the following table, fill in the purpose and expected effects of the drugs listed. We don't expect you to know them all, but some are common medications.

	Purpose	Expected effects	Contraindications	Consequences of incorrect use	Storage requirements	Disposal requirements
Paracetamol			Liver failure	Liver toxicity	Store in original packaging or Webster-Pak® at room temperature	Return to pharmacy to ensure environmentally safe disposal[1]
Frusemide			Previous allergy or adverse reaction to frusemide	Oedema or congestion may persist, or person may suffer dehydration	Store in original packaging or Webster-Pak® at room temperature	Return to pharmacy to ensure environmentally safe disposal[1]
Seretide (fluticasone/ salmeterol)			Previous allergy or adverse reaction to Seretide contents	Person may not be able to breathe properly or may suffer an asthma attack	Keep inhaler dry, and store at room temperature	Discard empty inhaler device into rubbish
Transiderm nitro patch			Dizziness or low blood pressure	Breakthrough chest pain	Store in foil packaging until ready to apply	Fold in half, sticky sides together, then place in rubbish
Insulin			Low blood sugar, or blood sugar level below level specified by the doctor	Poorly controlled diabetes	Store unopened insulin in the fridge. Store current supply at room temperature, protect from light and discard after 28 days	Dispose of needles and empty pens into sharps container. (Some insulin may remain in the pen.)
Pantoprazole			Person who needs their medications to be crushed – tablets cannot be crushed	Breakthrough symptoms of heartburn and indigestion	Store in original packaging or Webster-Pak® at room temperature	Return to pharmacy to ensure environmentally safe disposal[1]

Continued

211

	Purpose	Expected effects	Contraindications	Consequences of incorrect use	Storage requirements	Disposal requirements
Hydrozole cream clotrimazole/ hydrocortisone			Previous allergic reaction to clotrimazole or hydrocortisone; must not be applied to a bacterial infection or a shingles rash	Rash will not improve/ resolve	Store with lid on in a ziplock bag apart from other medications to prevent cross-contamination	Empty tubes can be placed in general rubbish. Return any partially used creams to pharmacy to ensure environmentally safe disposal[1]
Timoptol eye drops			Sensitivity to the preservative	Systemic side effects may occur, including dizziness, headache, bradycardia or wheezing	Store with lid on and discard one month after opening	Dispose of empty bottle into rubbish. Return any partially used bottles to pharmacy to ensure environmentally safe disposal[1]
Mylanta			Mylanta interacts with some medications. Always check with RN before administering.	Ongoing indigestion or, if given too much, person may get diarrhoea	Store unopened bottle at room temperature. Once bottle is open, store in fridge and discard after six months	Dispose of empty bottles into plastic recycling bin. Return any bottles with medication remaining to pharmacy to ensure environmentally safe disposal[1]
Risperdal Quicklet (risperidone)			Previous allergy or adverse reaction to risperidone	Persistent symptoms, drowsiness, dizziness	Store at room temperature in foil until immediately before use. Do not touch quicklets with your fingers	Return to pharmacy to ensure environmentally safe disposal[1]

[1]National Return and Disposal of Unwanted Medicines, www.health.gov.au/internet/main/publishing.nsf/Content/nmp-prescribers-return.htm. The National Return and Disposal of Unwanted Medicines, known as the RUM program, is a national not-for-profit company set up to enable consumers to return unwanted or out-of-date medicines to any pharmacy, at any time. The medicines returned are in no way reused or recycled. They are destroyed in an environmentally-friendly manner to avoid accidental childhood poisoning, medication misuse and toxic releases into the environment.

18. ASSISTING CLIENTS WITH THEIR MEDICATIONS: PROCEDURE

For your final assessment, you will be assessed at your workplace assisting clients with medication. You will go through the medication competencies set out in the appendix at the back of the 'Final Assessment' book in the classroom with your trainer/assessor and practise them prior to going out to the workplace.

Unit CHCCCS036:
Support relationships with carers and families

Table of Contents

INTRODUCTION

This workbook relates to the unit **CHCCCS036: Support relationships with carers and families**.

The workbook activities and final assessment tasks will enable you to:

- include carers and family members as part of the support team
- assess and respond to changes in the care relationship
- monitor and promote carer rights, health and wellbeing.

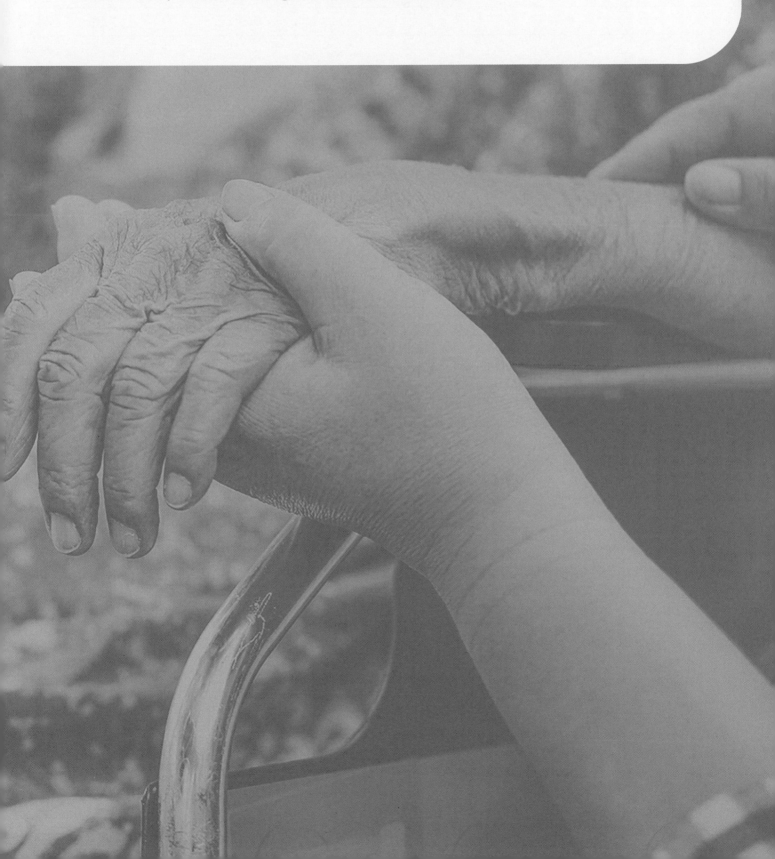

1. CARERS

_____

_____

_____

_____

_____

_____

_____

2. CONTEXT OF CARING IN AUSTRALIA

_____

_____

_____

_____

_____

_____

_____

_____

_____

_____

Culturally and linguistically diverse carers

_____

_____

_____

_____

_____

_____

_____

_____

_____

_____

_____

3. CARER LEGISLATION AND POLICY

_____
_____
_____
_____
_____
_____
_____
_____
_____
_____
_____
_____
_____
_____
_____
_____
_____
_____

4. MULTIDISCIPLINARY TEAMS

(pages 9–10 of Scott, Webb and Kostelnick, 5th edition)

_____
_____
_____
_____
_____

5. WORK ROLE BOUNDARIES FOR PAID SUPPORT WORKERS

_____
_____
_____
_____

6. INCLUDING CARERS AND FAMILY MEMBERS AS PART OF THE SUPPORT TEAM

_____
_____
_____
_____
_____

7. CARER SUPPORT

_____
_____
_____
_____
_____
_____
_____
_____

Activity 1

What things can carers do to keep healthy and take care of themselves?

_____
_____
_____
_____
_____
_____
_____

8. THE FAMILY CARING FOR A LOVED ONE WITH DEMENTIA

(page 401 of Scott, Webb and Kostelnick, 5th edition)

_____

_____

_____

_____

_____

_____

_____

_____

_____

_____

9. LIFE CYCLE TRANSITIONS AND HOW THIS CAN HAVE POSITIVE AND NEGATIVE IMPACTS ON THE CARER RELATIONSHIP WITH THE PERSON

_____

_____

_____

_____

_____

_____

_____

_____

10. CAREGIVER BURDEN

_____

_____

_____

_____

_____

11. RIGHTS AND ROLES OF DIFFERENT PEOPLE IN THE CARE RELATIONSHIP

_____

_____

_____

_____

_____

12. RESPONSIBILITIES OF DIFFERENT PEOPLE IN THE CARE RELATIONSHIP

_____

_____

_____

_____

_____

13. ASSESSING AND RESPONDING TO CHANGES IN THE CARE RELATIONSHIP

When caring for a family member, it is important to assess any physical or psychological risks to the carer and the person. What are some physical and psychological risks to the carer and the person?

_____

_____

_____

_____

_____

_____

_____

_____

Activity 2

Look at some of the risks that have been listed and outlined above. Choose one risk:

- How could you prevent this risk from occurring?
- If this risk occurs, what control measures can be put in place to eliminate or reduce the risks to the carer and person?

_____

_____

_____

_____

_____

_____

_____

_____

_____

_____

14. STRATEGIES FOR WORKING POSITIVELY WITH FAMILIES, CARERS AND FRIENDS IN RESIDENTIAL AGED CARE AND COMMUNITY SETTINGS

_____

_____

Carers' Health and Wellbeing

_____

_____

_____

_____

_____

_____

15. MONITORING AND PROMOTING CARER RIGHTS, HEALTH AND WELLBEING

_____

_____

_____

_____

_____

_____

_____

_____

_____

_____

16. ATTITUDES, STEREOTYPES AND MYTHS ASSOCIATED WITH CARING

_____

_____

_____

_____

_____

_____

_____